Ever Seen a Fat Fox?

Ever Seen a Fat Fox?

Human Obesity Explored

MIKE GIBNEY

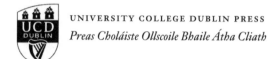

UNIVERSITY COLLEGE DUBLIN PRESS
Preas Choláiste Ollscoile Bhaile Átha Cliath

First published 2016
by University College Dublin Press
UCD Humanities Institute, Room H103
Belfield
Dublin 4
Ireland
www.ucdpress.ie

ISBN 978-1-910820-08-7 pb

Cataloguing in Publication data
available from the British Library

The right of Mike Gibney to be identified
as the authors of this work has been asserted by him

Typeset in Scotland in Adobe Garamond,
Janson and Trade Gothic by Ryan Shiels
Text design by Lyn Davies
Printed in England on acid-free paper by
CPI Antony Rowe, Chippenham, Wiltshire

For Jo

Contents

Acknowledgements and Declarations

I am extremely grateful to those who read and commented on technical aspects of earlier drafts: Aifric O'Sullivan, Aideen McKevitt, Greg Foley, Marianne Walsh, Julie Dowsett, Eileen Gibney and my sister Rosemary. A particular thanks is due to Professor Ciaran Forde of the Singapore Institute of Clinical Sciences who applied his critical eye on the food intake regulation chapter, an area where I'm a tad out of depth. Again I thank the staff at UCD Press, Noelle Moran and Damien Lynam, for their fantastic help, patience and encouragement in getting this project to market. Thanks to Daniel and Sarah in Origin Design, Dublin, for the illustration and cover design, to Ryan Shiels, Scotland, for his skilled typesetting, and to Peter O'Connell for publicity. Finally I would like to thank all my friends and family who encouraged me along and who made so many useful suggestions. Of these, my wife Jo, to whom this book is dedicated, has helped so much with her encouragement and patience and not least in getting all the final details right.

I include this declaration of interests in the spirit that guides the norms and values that shape integrity in scientific research. During the writing of this book, I served on advisory committees for Nestlé's Research Centre (remunerated), for Cereal Partners Worldwide (remunerated), both in Switzerland, Google's Food Innovation Lab (non-remunerated) in the US and the Nutrition Panel of the Sackler Institute of the New York Academy of Sciences (non-remunerated). I am chair of the Board of the Food Safety Authority of Ireland (remunerated) in Dublin and I'm a board member of the European branch of the International Life Sciences Institute (non-remunerated) in Brussels. My final major research project on personalised nutrition (www.food4me.org) as Principal Investigator involved the following companies: Phillips Electronics (Eindhoven and Cambridge), Crème Software (Dublin), DSM (Basel), Bio-Sense (Brussels), NuGO (Wageningen) and Vitas (Oslo).

Preface

Most people would be accepting of the following narrative to briefly describe the main issues facing the globe with respect to excess weight and specifically obesity: the modern epidemic of obesity started in the mid-1970s to mid-1980s in the US, and was quickly followed by similar growth surges in the prevalence of obese persons across the globe, which, to this day, continues to rise almost everywhere. As the prevalence of overweight and obesity rises in a given country there is a parallel rise in a number of adverse health outcomes, most notably, high blood pressure, adult onset (type 2) diabetes and heart disease. The scale of obesity, ranked by the WHO as the fifth leading cause of death globally,[1] is estimated in the US to cost just over $92,000 per obese person per lifetime amounting presently to $20 trillion.[2]

The rising levels of obesity are associated, and I stress associated, with an abundance of widely advertised cheap food and beverages, mainly industrially processed and high in sugar, fat and salt. Physical activity, which in itself is very healthy, plays a moderate role in weight gain and weight loss. Caloric balance is what matters. Governments can help tackle obesity through taxation of bad foods or the restriction of bad food availability in or near schools and by many other regulatory means. But ultimately, weight management is the responsibility of each individual. Some people blame their genes but the reality is that human genes have remained constant for dozens of millennia while our environment and the availability of cheap, industrially produced foods has soared. Obesity, in a sense, is the new tobacco. Large companies get rich on poor quality, even addictive foods and are in denial of any responsibility.[3] Until their power is curbed with taxes, until cheap food product promotion and availability is restricted and until powerful and shocking images are displayed to the obese, the obesity epidemic will continue to grow, particularly among the most vulnerable such as all children and the socially disadvantaged.

So, do I agree with the above? If the answer were unequivocally 'yes' then, clearly, I wouldn't have written this book. So, let's ask the converse question: 'Do I comprehensively deny the general truth of this narrative?' The answer to that is also 'no'. I fully accept that overweight and obesity together represent one of the most important and challenging areas facing global public health nutrition, that excess body weight is a global pandemic and rapidly rising in the emerging economies, that it is a major contributor to non-communicable diseases such as diabetes, hypertension and heart disease and that it is a major drain on national health service costs. Among these points that I don't dispute at the high level, I challenge the way in which they are grossly oversimplified by populist advocates who parade them as such in the media and who lay them out to policy makers for implementation. I do question the simple concept that the modern food industry is to blame, I absolutely dispute the rejection of a role for genes in deciding who gets obese and I do not see obesity as the new tobacco of public health. In addition to all of these, I see some key issues that are quietly ignored at the policy level such as eating disorders, the stigmatisation of the overweight and the fatal flaw of epidemiology and public health in not embracing a sympathetic feeling for the individuals that make up the populations they study and their every joys and woes. I also believe that governments pay lip service to obesity. They allow big egos to shape obesity-related policy when in fact it is the moral duty of government to do so. They allow the simplistic view of obesity to become the hobby of governmental aficionados from Michelle Obama[4] to New York's Mayor Bloomberg.[5] And all the time, they keep their hands in their pockets.

Quite simply, the full picture is very complicated and the problem that advocates face in communicating complex messages to the general public and to policy makers is that they must simplify the complicated and they must continually repeat the simplified message until it becomes a given that only contrarian and sceptical luddites like myself or vested industrial interests would challenge. It is against this background that I wrote this book. I hope that by the end of this book, the reader will look back on this narrative and understand it better. I don't ask them to dismiss this narrative or to radically re-write it. But maybe in casual conversation they might be in a better position to express opinions that are a little more open to doubt than is generally the case at present. The objective of this book is not to solve the problem, but in analysing it, to inform the reader of its complexity.

A quick overview of the book is as follows: the first few chapters look at the manner in which we define obesity, how we use those measures to gauge its health impact and how we measure the major input of calories as everyday foods. These chapters are intended to be informative but, as in keeping with the overall philosophy of this book, the basic tenets outlined in it will be challenged. Even though serious flaws will be identified with all of them, the book adopts a conservative view and seeks to live with what we have. We then move to two chapters which probe the history of obesity and the history of the food chain because a popular but very incorrect view is that these went pear shaped just recently, in the last half millennium for example, leading to our present problem with obesity. This is not the case. We have always had obesity as long as we had affluence and the modern 'processed food' industry dates back millennia. The Greeks used crystalline sugar at the turn of the tenth century and Aztec girls danced adorned with popcorn garlands half a millennium ago.

The next few chapters focus on the present day dietary supply of foods and nutrients. They follow the rise and fall and rise again of fashions in the meaning-less but nonetheless extremely popular quest for the super calories. They look at the drivers of food choice and deliberately ignore, well almost so, the brain and focus primarily on our obesogenic environment and how some of us manage to cope with that while others have difficulty in so doing and this section also looks at how our genes shape this variation in how we respond to a calorie-laden food supply. Of course, this part of the book must also look at the opposite end of the calorie equation: its disposal as energy through physical activity. It will make the point that a sedentary lifestyle is a killer every bit if not bigger than obesity but it manages to be its poor relation. Before moving to people and the problem in its causes and solutions, a few minor but important inputs are discussed, some of which receive great media attention while others don't.

People come next – the skinny persons with anorexia nervosa and the many with other awful eating disorders. If these lie at one end of a scale of human concern, the obese lie at the other, scorned for their failure to act responsibly, detested by many in society and utterly stigmatised for their disgusting grossness. But if the fatties and their bigots deserve the microscope of integrity, others also do: non-governmental organisations, global organisations, scientists, the media, editors of scientific journals and the food industry are all called to account for their upholding of scientific integrity and they all do badly. And so we then come to the crunch of the book: what is to be done? What should individuals do, how should governments behave and how should society act to tackle the phenomenon of overweight and obesity? By then the reader will have explored the full spectrum of relevant issues, in a manner that explains and criticises but always leaves a way forward.

In the writing of this book, many have queried my chosen title *Ever Seen a Fat Fox?*; so let me explain my reasoning. Humans are the only species that get fat. We and the fox can develop many common cancers or diseases of the gut or heart. Each species can suffer parasitic, bacterial and viral infections. We each can injure a limb and suffer traumatic injuries. But foxes, like all feral animals, don't develop lifelong obesity leading to major illnesses from diabetes to hypertension. Humans have a unique relationship with food that neither the fox nor any other species has. We share food, not just with immediate kin, but also with total strangers. Foxes don't. Modern humans do not procure their own food *ab initio*. Foxes do. We live in highly complex and ever changing environments where technological innovation plays an enormous role and where we divide labour from the procurement of food to its processing, transport, storage, distribution and cooking. Foxes don't. We communicate in the most advanced ways through traditional media and now social media. Foxes have very limited communication and live solely within their own species. It is to me blindingly obvious that, notwithstanding a common sharing of most of our genomes with animals, we are fat because we organised society in such a way as to make that not simply possible, but probable. That being the case, we can dream that the trillions of dollars spent on reductionist biology will one day lead to a miracle cure à la drug route such that we can continue to lead our lives as we do and kiss obesity goodbye. Dream on I say. Obesity is so complex from both a social and biological perspective that we will make slow progress in our understanding of bits and pieces of the biological jigsaw and even slower progress in the social jigsaw. In the meantime we can wait and hope. Or we can recognise that obesity is simply a consequence of the way we live and we can seek to change our ways. It's no easy road and that is the central tenet of this book: beware of self-serving advocates selling simple solutions. Good luck if you think that they will work. So, the not so fat fox is my inspiration for how we should see the challenge of human obesity.

MIKE GIBNEY
Dublin, April 2016

Abbreviations

AIDS	Acquired Immune Deficiency Syndrome
ANRED	Anorexia Nervosa and Related Eating Disorders
BBC	British Broadcasting Corporation
BMI	Body Mass Index
BMJ	*British Medical Journal*
CD	Caloric Density
CIA	Central Intelligence Agency
CLA	Conjugated Linoleic Acid
CV	Curriculum Vitae
DEXA	Dual-Energy X-Ray Absorptiometry
DNA	Deoxyribonucleic Acid
DSM	*Diagnostic and Statistical Manual of Mental Disorders*
ECG	Electrocardiogram
ED-NOS	Eating Disorders Not Otherwise Specified
EF	Enjoyment of Food
ENGOs	Environmental Non-Governmental Organisations
EPODE	Ensemble Prévenons l'Obesité Des Enfants
EU	European Union
FBI	*Federal Bureau of Investigation*
FDA	Food and Drug Administration
FTO	Fat Mass and Obesity Associated (Gene)
GRADE	Grading of Recommendations, Assessment, Development and Evaluation
HFCS	High Fructose Corn Syrup
HIV	Human Immunodeficiency Virus
HMSO	Her Majesty's Stationary Office
IQ	Intelligence Quotient
LG	Lucky Goldstar
MD	Medicinae Doctor
METS	Metabolic Equivalent of a Task
MGI	McKinsey Global Institute

MGM	Metro-Goldwyn Mayer
MLI	Metropolitan Life Insurance
MRI	Magnetic Resonance Imaging
NEAT	Non-Exercise Activity Thermogenesis
NIH	National Institute of Health
NGOs	Non-Governmental Organisations
PKU	Phenylketonuria
PWS	Prader-Willi Syndrome
SMART	Specific, Measurable, Attainable, Realistic and Time-Bound
SMEs	Small and Medium Enterprises
SNP	Single Nucleotide Polymorphism
SRSE	Satiety Responsiveness – Slow Eating
SSBs	Sugar-Sweetened Beverages
TAF	Trim and Fit
TB	Tuberculosis
UK	United Kingdom
UN	United Nations
UNICEF	United Nations International Children's Emergency Fund
US	United States
USDA	United States Department of Agriculture
VAS	Visual Analog Scale
WHO	World Health Organization
WHR	Waist-to-Hip Ratio
YFAS	Yale Food Addiction Score
ZTE	Zhong Xing Telecommunication Equipment

CHAPTER ONE

Ever Seen a Fat Fox?

In the course of a harsh winter, a fox becomes thinner and thinner until he fears that he will starve. One day he comes across food inside a hollow tree, this having been hidden there by a man who believes the hole in the trunk to be too small for an animal to enter. The fox can get through the hole having become so thin. He eats all the food, but finds himself too fat to get out. He has to wait for a few days until he is thin again before he can get out again. (*Aesop's Fables*, 'The too fat fox')

With the exception of domestic pets, some experimental animals and some farmed stock, man is the only species that develops obesity. Some animal species gain fat when food is abundant and lose it when the winter comes and food is scarce. Unlike man, all of the animals in these species gain and lose fat when appropriate. But it remains a fact: we alone manage to develop overweight and obesity and it is only by the hand of humans that any other species becomes fat. A fox will eat sufficient food, and no more than that, to meet the energy needs of procreation, the procurement of food and the protection of its lair. Apparently, we share most of our genes with the fox. We have genes the fox doesn't need such as the genes for speech and language. However, the fox expresses far more genes than we do in those attributes of importance in hunting – the genes for the senses of sight, sound and smell. When we move up the evolutionary chain to our nearest neighbours, the great apes, we share even more of our genes with these animals, but again, they don't get obese. Foxes and apes digest, absorb and metabolise fat and glucose just like us and we share common hormones that regulate metabolism and regulate the control of food intake. But you've never seen a fat fox.

To understand obesity, its origins and its management, we must look beyond the biology to the social dimension of our world. Literally, billions of dollars and euros per year are invested in obesity research through private and state funding. The vast majority of this spend is on the minutia of the regulation of energy balance and in the majority of instances we use animals to study this minutia because we can conduct experiments on such animals that would not be considered ethical in humans. Such experiments can tell us a great deal about the metabolic pathways that lead to the accumulation of excess fat and we can be confident that when we see an obese person, we can explain in detail how things happened in terms of biochemical and metabolic events and how our nutrients were absorbed, transformed, transported, stored, released and oxidised for energy. We can explain the links between key organs from body fat, the gut, muscle and the liver right up to the brain, in the developing pathology of excess body fat. But we cannot avoid what is glaringly obvious. All who are overweight and obese have persisted for lengthy periods in consuming more calories by way of food and drink than they have expended in terms of energy. They have also done so involuntarily, except in rare cases. So human alone overeats. If we share so many genes with all the other animal species that don't gain weight on a permanent basis, then we should be looking beyond complex biological pathways to understand obesity. Why do people overeat and why do they opt for an increasingly sedentary lifestyle? This is a very complex question and this book will seek to explore that complexity and to make the case that the so-called 'battle' against obesity can only be solved by a multi-level, multi-disciplinary approach, adequately funded by central governments and within a framework for action that has a long-term view. The present chapter explores the complex nature of modern human civilisation and how it might both contribute to obesity and at the same time determine the success of otherwise well-meaning plans to tackle the obesity question.

Homo sapiens: Uniquely Wise and Uniquely Fat

Life on earth is about 4.5 billion years old. The first 2.5 billion years of this life consisted of single-cell organisms and about one billion years later, multi-cell organisms in the form of marine sponges arrived. Half a billion years later we saw the first animals emerge from the sea and the first *hominins* arrived just seven million years ago. During all this time, genes ruled. Everything that each species needed for life and death was in their genes. As recently as 160,000–200,000 years ago something remarkable happened when evolution saw a competitor to genetic rule arrive. Humans learned to do something that no other species had achieved. They had acquired the capacity to learn from one another and to share ideas.[1] The capacity to transmit knowledge through rudimentary baby-like grunts and sign language meant that the capacity not just to survive but to develop to a higher plane was now significantly independent of genetic data. The rate of development of the human race would take off. Animals can learn and can be very smart. Thus a crow, given access to a pile of stones and a peanut floating in a bottle of water, as yet inaccessible to the crow, will learn to place the stones in the bottle until the level of the water rises to let the crow have access to the succulent peanut as it gradually floats to the top. Smart crow. However, each crow has to learn this individually. Humans alone transmit knowledge from one to another. Richard Dawkins, in his famous book *The Selfish Gene*, coins the term meme (pronounced as in cream) to cover the transmission of ideas, knowledge and concepts across society.[2] The concept of memes may have its challengers but it does help us to understand some aspects of human communication. Memes are what define culture and culture is what defines humanity. Foxes don't have memes. Foxes don't have culture.

Both genes and memes are what Dawkins call 'replicators'. We inherit our genes from our parents and depending on the lottery of life, those parents from whom we obtained our genes might live in Dublin, Dubai, Denver, Dar es Salaam, Dubrovnik, Durban or Delhi. The human baby is unique in its early life with a very strong dependence on its parents. The young fox is up and about and ready for life within hours of birth. Its requirements for life are hardwired into their brain with very little left to learn other than where home is. Its life is almost entirely determined by the gene replicator. In contrast, the newborn baby must learn the language and culture of the society into which it was born. It must learn the norms, the manners, the rituals, the loves, the fears and the hates of its society. In time it will learn how to play its role in that society all of which will be driven by the meme replicator. The gene replicator will still be there to regulate the digestion and metabolism of food, to manage the details of its reproductive needs, to manage its immune system, its vision, its smell, its physique, its looks and all its basic biological needs. But almost everything that is important in its society and culture is meme replicated. Foxes don't do memes.

As genetic variation arose in the history of man, some conferred such an advantage that the gene replicator persisted. In other instances, the gene replicator was made redundant. Consider, for example, the gene for the synthesis of vitamin C. It no longer exists in vertebrates because there is plenty of vitamin C around in foods. Why waste our energy making the vitamin when it abounds in nature's supermarkets? Similarly memes must find a permanent place in society or else fade away and die, redundant to the needs of man's progress. Remember the ice-bucket challenge that swept the world in 2014? That was a meme but it's not a meme to stay. The practice of growing a moustache by men in November for charity, the 'Movember' meme, has persisted but it's not likely to be here in a decade's time. But the meme for fire capture, for cooking, for social dining, for music, art, song and so on, these memes are forever. Genes may explain the neurological networks of the joy of music. But there is no music gene. Memes are part and parcel of human culture. Foxes don't do culture. They don't have rock festivals, the Olympic Games, high mass, opera, air travel, the internet, language, competitive sport or anything resembling human culture. Not even the higher order primates scratch the surface in achieving human civilisation. Memes drive our attitudes to food and body weight regulation: the Atkins Diet, the South Beach Diet, the Grapefruit Diet, the Paleo Diet, the 3 Day Diet, the super foods from quinoa to kale to berries and smoothies. These are all meme-spread drivers of human behaviour toward weight control. They are fostered *ad nauseam* by the mass media and form the latest opinions of television and social media food gurus. They pedal nonsense memes that lead us to 'detoxification', to 'fat melting' to 'fast metabolism'. They promote pills, herbal teas, fat removing wearable devices and physical workouts. As we will see toward the latter part of this book, memes spread the latest scientific findings that hit the headlines and confuse the general public. Memes bring us the fashions of food and health: out with fat as the villain – in with sugar. An understanding of obesity in modern human culture needs to be aware of these drivers.

Nutrition: Religion and Mysticism Both Past and Present

In his very scholarly work entitled *Sapiens: A Brief History of Humankind*,[3] Yuval Harari makes some important points which add to the role of memes in shaping modern culture. He makes the point that the ability of early humans to transmit such knowledge as 'there is a lion down by the estuary' or 'there are lots of salmon at the rock pools' was important beyond belief in distinguishing man from beasts but it was not enough. Man was to rapidly evolve very strong social ties and thus social gossip was every bit as vital as the location of predators or food. As he puts it himself: 'It is not enough for men and women to know the whereabouts of lions and bison. It's much more important for them to know who in their band hates whom, who is sleeping with whom, who is honest and who is a cheat.' That group-binding sharing of gossip is still as important today. However, Harari argues that something happened when the size of the social circle increased such that gossip was fine in the finite structures of clan-like groups but not for large tribes. It was not that we stopped communicating about lions, salmon and bison and it was not that we stopped gossiping. We now invented 'the ability to transmit information about things that do not exist at all'. These included legends, myths, gods and religions. These never bothered foxes. In her book *A Case for God*, Karen Armstrong takes this further in separating 'mythos' from 'logos'.[4] The latter was beyond debate: the sun rose in the east, winter was cold, young people generally grew to be adults, if pricked we bled and so on. That was logos. On the other hand mythos was about what we couldn't explain: Why were there no rains this year? Why have we had floods two years in a row? Why have so many bison come our way this year? Why do some babies die? Why do some old people never suffer before death while others are tormented, presumably by demons? These questions can all be framed such as to be answered in the myths, legends and religions that man developed. And food issues played a huge role in mythology and in religious service. Group sacrifices of highly desired gastronomic treats such as fatted calves are legendary in religious lore and personal sacrifices of denial exist in every religion from the Christian Lenten fast to the Muslim Ramadan fasts. To deviate from normal behaviour in relation to food was sinful and this brings us to the moral stance of society on obesity. There are seven deadly sins in certain Christian faiths of which three might be regarded as 'cerebral' (pride, wrath and envy) with four involving what we call today 'lifestyle choices': gluttony and greed associated with diet, sloth associated with a sedentary lifestyle and of course lust associated with sex. Food was the perfect illustration of the need to balance pleasure and sin and so great was the former and so dire the latter in its consequences that the concept of asceticism evolved with hermits living lives of great self-sacrifice, effectively taking total control of their body in terms of food, exercise and sex, so that their body (effectively detached from 'them') could not get in the way of the pursuit of the moral ideal. Gluttony was by far the most visible of the seven deadly sins and it was gluttony that attracted most attention from those seeking the afterlife. As ever, the organised churches had very profound views on gluttony, none more so than Pope Gregory the Great who managed to define six levels of gluttony: 'nimis (eating too much), ardenter (eating with unbecoming eagerness), forente (eating wildly), praepropere (not waiting until decent mealtimes), laute (enjoying food that is too expensive) and studiose (being too picky)'. Food and religion remained inextricably linked right up to the twentieth century when men like John Harvey Kellogg linked a healthy diet to the avoidance of excessive sex. So when man separated from other species including at an early stage our friend the fox, the path to mysticism and a role for diet therein was constructed. Today however, that apparently useful bond is all but gone. Religion is in decline and in its place come others waving myths and anecdotes. All are designed to help us to give sustenance to that inner self that once we nourished with religion. Today, we nourish that inner self with antioxidants, super foods, colonic irrigation, fasting and multivitamins. We balance ying and yang. We follow today's guru with tomorrow's and we collectively fool ourselves that our inner wellbeing can be nourished such that our organs will flourish to elegant longevity. We are a meme-dominated society when it comes to diet and health and that is partly due to human desperation to explain our ancient 'mythos', whether it is the Hunza diet of the Khyber Pass or spirulina, a micro-alga of the Aztecs. When we come to look at diet and health, to weight and physical activity management, we need to understand that the drivers or memes of modern man are rarely our allies.

Ambivalence: A Uniquely Human Condition

The average urban fox is no longer scared of cars, of sirens, of house alarms, security lighting or even our pet dogs. A fox can spot a perceived hazard and can find a way to negate it or to get around it, although sometimes the fox doesn't survive. But if the fox survives, it can recall that hazard and deal with it in a way that doesn't threaten its life. But foxes don't imagine dreadful hazards. Humans certainly do. The Ebola viral epidemic scares people. Obesity doesn't. The public is by and large immune to the constant drip of media coverage of the many putative causes and dire consequences of obesity. But Ebola is still a headline to heed. Three factors operate simultaneously to stir fear in the public.[5] The threat should be unfamiliar, dreaded and largely beyond ones control. Ebola hits all three. But obesity doesn't for we are all familiar with it, it isn't really dreaded, and by and large we can always manage our weight if we have to. But obesity is actually a greater epidemic than that of Ebola. The annual death rate from obesity is estimated at 2.8 million while at the time of writing just under 11,300 people have contracted the Ebola virus, almost a 250-fold difference. To redress this imbalance of human concern between threats to health that are widely feared but of low global magnitude and those which are socially tolerated but of high global magnitude, we need to try and move the consumer from an emotional analysis of public health to a more logical analysis. We need to describe the scale, the costs and the consequences of obesity and hope that this might re-frame how it is that society views obesity. It is, I'm afraid, a long shot. The science of risk assessment has known for many years that the fears people have about the human food chain are emotionally driven and, as such, are largely immune to logical arguments. But some hopefully will listen and learn.

On a global scale, the economic costs of obesity are on a par with the health care costs arising from smoking or the health care consequences arising from the combined effects of violent crime, terrorism and warfare. On a national basis, the UK health care costs of obesity equal the combined total costs of its police service, fire service, prison service and its law courts.[6] Ebola infection will be conquered as was HIV and several virulent flu strains. Obesity has to be addressed but it raises challenges not apparent in other public health care areas. Thus smoking is a single issue, which allows for a highly focused and well-funded campaign to effectively eliminate tobacco from society. Similarly, road traffic accident rates are targeted through better cars, better roadways and better driver behaviour. Obesity has to be tackled from the supply side of the food chain and through behavioural change. Strategies to achieve these ends abound, each championed by some interest group or another, but until the political will exists, as it does for tobacco control and road traffic accidents, the epidemic of obesity will prevail and its ranking in the spectrum of society's great fears will remain low. In addition to the logic of economic costs, we can also move to the argument of the global scale of obesity.

The Global World of Homo Sapiens

Humans alone wandered the world settling in far-flung regions from the frozen tundra to the sun-scorched deserts, from the rain forests to the great plains. Everywhere that humans went, human civilisation took root and with it all of our trade, culture and know-how. The advent of global travel, global trade and global communications meant that all corners of the world had access to more or less the same market, be it Armani jeans, Ray-Ban sunglasses or an affordable modern food chain. Moreover, global trade meant growth in local economies such that the average spending power rose globally and with it the lifestyle of the modern world. Inevitably, that also meant obesity, and in large numbers. Like any epidemic, obesity has spread to all corners of the globe but to different levels and at different rates. The McKinsey Global Institute's (MGI) report on obesity shows that countries such as Hong Kong, South Korea and Japan share the same level of obesity (5–15%) as China, Malaysia and Thailand but are on average ten times wealthier.[7] Undoubtedly, this is caused by recent mass urbanisation in China, Malaysia and Thailand. On the other hand these same three countries, Hong Kong, South Korea and Japan, share the same average wealth as the US, UK and Australia and yet have much lower rates of obesity (30–5%). This difference is more likely due to an adherence to a traditional Asian diet. Given that approximately eight cities the size of Chicago are created every year, mostly in China, and that migration to urban centres can adversely affect both lifestyle and food choice, wealth is probably a very important driver of obesity. Increasing personal wealth is essential for the poorer sections of society to invest in the welfare of their children through better health care and better education, which in turn brings with it greater economic independence and social freedom. Within countries, the epidemic also varies with higher obesity rates generally, but not always seen, among the lower socio-economic groups. Gender also plays a role with much higher levels of obesity in women in many countries, particularly among Arab states and the Caribbean and Pacific islands. Although developed countries have a four-fold higher obesity rate than developing countries, the growth in rates of obesity over the last three decades is five times higher in developing countries. All in all, obesity is one of the greatest global public health challenges we face today and of all comparable challenges, it is by far the most complex to resolve.

Whatever Makes You Happy?

If the ordinary citizen has difficulty in understanding the grave concerns of nutritional epidemiology and public health nutrition, is it possible that an opposite flow of understanding is necessary? When epidemiologists describe the gross landscape of lifestyle and obesity, they are data-driven and operate solely at the level of the population. They set the scene for public health nutritionists to advise governments and health agencies on how to tackle obesity at the national and local level. But they do not sit down with the obese and overweight to understand their everyday concerns. And as we will see, these everyday concerns of family, of spouses, of children and grandchildren, of work, of finance, of homes, of leisure, of dreams and hopes, all of these shape how individuals think about food and health. These don't enter the world of epidemiology or public health nutrition and it is to these everyday concerns of ordinary citizens that we turn next.

Cats purr and dogs sleep at our feet, clear and obvious signs of content-ment. Presumably, foxes also can exhibit contentment. But no animal species can match humans for the complexity of their contentment and happiness and to understand the social dimension of human obesity we really do need to delve a little into the science of human happiness and in doing so, I draw heavily on Professor Paul Dolan's book, *Finding Happiness by Design*.[8] The original thinkers on happiness focused on the balance between pleasure and pain. You were happiest if you had very little negativity (pain) and lots of positivity (pleasure). A more recent aspect of happiness replaces the balance of the enjoyment–suffering axis with a different axis, that of purpose–pointlessness. The former is associated with positive feelings such as fulfilment, meaning and worthwhileness, while the latter is associated with boredom and futility. This pleasure–purpose principle is central to the interpretation of human happiness as outlined by Professor Dolan. Happiness is not simply about pleasure. It is also about purpose. In large surveys, people are asked to rate various activities on a scale of one (low) to six (high) as regards the pleasure they give them and the extent to which they give them purpose in their lives. Work scores high on purpose but very low on pleasure. Television viewing is the exact opposite: high on pleasure and low on purpose. Eating is just below television viewing for pleasure but moves quite up the scale on purpose. Thus people find eating highly pleasurable but they also find it mildly purposeful since they are aware of the needs to abate hunger and hopefully to do so overall in a healthy manner. If eating is high on the pleasure scale, where does excess body weight fit on both the pleasure and purpose scales? To understand the links between obesity and happiness, we must first learn about the drivers of happiness. These can be as diverse as our love lives, our financial circumstances, family, our looks and image, our ambitions, our cares, our self-belief, our self-esteem, our health and wellbeing, careers, children, ageing parents and whatever makes you happy or unhappy. The process of producing happiness requires us to allocate our attention to these drivers of happiness. Attention, the happiness experts tell us, is a finite resource and thus attention spent on one driver of pleasure or purpose means less attention is spent on other such drivers. According to the research of Professor Paul Dolan, there are two ways to maintain happiness once one has gained weight. The first is to lose the weight. That will return you to normal and make you happy. The second is to adopt the 'so what?' attitude. Dieting comes with a relentless day-in, day-out mental effort that we can see all around us and largely leads to a temporary loss of weight with most people bouncing right back to their fat weight after that holiday or wedding or whatever seemed a good reason to lose weight at the time. Why not just live with your obesity and devote that mental effort to more productive drivers of happiness be it work or golf or gardening or the church or whatever. All of Professor Dolan's research shows that it is the second option that will dominate. Everyone around them is overweight so what's the issue? Health is not a problem now but job security, love life, ageing parents, income, children, neighbours are all more deserving of immediate attention.

The Nobel laureate in economics, Daniel Kahneman, in his book *Thinking Fast and Slow* describes our decision-making processes in two systems.[9] System 1 he argues: 'operates automatically and quickly, with little or no effort and no sense of voluntary control.' In contrast, System 2 requires attention and involves 'effortful mental activities'. It involves concentration and choice. So let's spend a while understanding System 1 and System 2. Consider a bank teller engaged all morning in monetary transactions, which require knowledge, thought and mental effort. That is System 2 (effortful mental activities). Then at lunch time, the teller enjoys the company of his or her friends and the chat turns to issues such as sport, politics, fashion, books and so on. Views are expressed but mostly these views are gut feelings, instincts, and intuition and are based more on superficial reflection than deep analysis requiring serious mental effort. You either like George Clooney or you don't and nobody expects a detailed analysis of your views on Mr Clooney. All of this lunch time banter is System 1 (automatic and rapid decisions).

Attention to drivers of happiness can be managed by these two conceptual systems that operate our brainpower. There was a famous experiment carried out at Harvard in which basketball teams in black or in white sports gear played a match.[10] The researchers took a video and asked subjects to accurately count the number of times that the ball was passed by the white team. When the test was over, they were asked if there was anything out of the way they had noticed or any participants other than the players. A total of 50% of the subjects failed to spot a person dressed as a gorilla strolling across the court in the middle of the video. When they were shown it again, the 50% who hadn't spotted the gorilla couldn't believe how they had missed this event. But they had. What this showed is that when your mind is focused on System 2 (counting passes of the basketball), something as simple as the interloping gorilla (a simple System 1 observation: that's a gorilla) was missed by half the population. To understand System 1 and food we need to turn to a simple study which flashed images past people such that their System 1 automatically and unconsciously noted them, without any role for the mental effort aspects of System 2.[11] One set of images was of fast food. The other was of plain squares. Those shown the subliminal fast food pictures subsequently read a set text 15 seconds faster than those shown the squares. Fast food has connotations with snappy, quick eating, more to achieve purpose than pleasure. So when subliminally exposed to images of fast food from big-brand suppliers, that snappy frame of mind determined utterly unrelated behaviour. Other studies look at a related phenomenon the 'spillover effect'. This relates what you do and see to other unrelated events. For example, people exposed to videos of exercise subsequently eat more when offered a snack than those shown control neutral videos. Another example asked students to step on and off a box for two minutes.[12] They were divided into four groups: Group 1 received ten pence per step; Group 2 received two pence per step; Group 3 did not receive any financial reward but received strong encouragement to continue stepping; Group 4 received neither financial nor verbal encouragement. Groups 1 and 2 did 105 steps and Groups 3 and 4 did 95 steps. They were the objective measures. But how did they feel? Groups 1 and 3 were most satisfied with their performance. They all agreed that the two minutes of work expended about 20–30 calories. But then the twist came. After the test and on their own, the students were offered a free selection of snacks and sandwiches. Groups 1 and 3 consumed 320 calories compared to Groups 2 and 4 who consumed 240 calories. Groups 1 and 3 were happier with themselves and that happiness spilled over into allowing them to eat more. This happens in real life every day and many examples exist in the scientific literature to support these findings. These are extremely complex social behaviours that go beyond the claims that this or that food causes obesity by this or that complex biological pathway. The fox forages on whatever food it might find in our suburban bin and processes it along those same biological pathways. But it eats no more than it needs to live, as it must. Once again, with the exception of Aesop's fabled fox, you've never seen a fat fox. Happiness research tells us that we balance pleasure and purpose by applying attention to their drivers and that attention devoted to one driver reduces the attention devoted to another. A recent UK study has thrown direct light on the link between happiness and body weight.[13] The National Childhood Measurement Programme records weight and height of children four to five and ten to eleven years old. This anti-obesity programme provides parents with a standardised written feedback. A survey of randomly selected parental responses to feedback from this programme showed that the majority of parents rejected the suggestion that their child had a health issue because of excess weight. The parents believed that 'health and happiness was more important than weight'. We shall see through this book that well-meant intervention does not take into account the holistic picture, of which happiness is primary.[13]

From the Fox to the Human

Dietary advice to populations cannot be written on blank sheets. The sheets are in fact already adorned with many constraints, constraints that are part and parcel of the way we live. So like it or not, when we set out on public health nutrition campaigns, the issues seem sensible and logical to those who draft them. But research shows that humans manage their happiness in terms of pleasure and purpose by devoting attention to where the biggest happiness dividends will be found and part of that happiness is driven by our environmental cues and by spill over effects of one healthy action on another unhealthy action. Fears of hazards such as Ebola are real but readily forgotten. So too are the logic of the dire global health consequences of obesity. They are noted and then conveniently parked. Not lost, just parked. Changing human behaviour is complex and must take account of what might be done by individuals and what might be done by society to facilitate change. Both are needed. Foxes don't have the level of social and economic organisation that humans have and thus they don't get fat. For them, fatness would be a big disadvantage. For humans, obesity is a massive public health problem, inextricably linked to a poorly understood social dimension and operated by an increasingly understood biological dimension. It shouldn't surprise us that with human fatness being such a complex issue, that our understanding of it is imperfect or indeed that the tools we use to measure and tackle it have significant shortcomings. It is to the overall complexity of human obesity that we now turn.

CHAPTER TWO

Obesity: Measurements and Metrics

Most people will know someone who had a consultation with medical specialties such as neurology, gastroenterology or cardiology. However, nobody makes an appointment to see an epidemiologist because this branch of medicine deals with population health rather than individual health. Modern day epidemiology can be traced back to Dr John Snow, who disconnected the tap from the water pump in Broad Street London, thereby ending a cholera outbreak.[1] Of the 71 deaths Snow investigated, 61 were of people living in the vicinity of Broad Street and thus users of the pump. Three deaths occurred in children who lived nearer another pump but who went to school close to the Broad Street pump. Five others 'preferred' the water at Broad Street over their local pump. Only two deaths could not be linked to the guilty pump. All of this happened prior to our understanding of infective bacteria such as cholera. And so, armed with a dot map and his 71 case histories, the pump was disabled. Clearly, Snow could not have had definitive proof of cause and effect and so he acted based on statistical probability and in doing so, he saved many lives. In modern epidemiology, there are two main causes of population ill health that are studied. First there are infectious diseases such as HIV, Ebola, polio, tuberculosis, smallpox and the like. These are referred to as acute conditions because the actual symptoms rapidly follow infection. The second area of study for modern epidemiology is in chronic disease where the agent is non-infective and where the symptoms arise long after exposure. The relationship between smoking and lung cancer is one example. Another is that between high blood pressure and stroke. Obesity and its adverse effects fall into this category where the adverse effect is most frequently implicated by statistical data. One cannot do a clinical trial to verify by experiment that smoking is associated with a higher incidence of lung cancer. That would be unethical. However, in human nutrition, dietary intervention trials can be conducted and can confirm or refute the putative association, inferred from epidemiological probability, between some dietary pattern and the disease in question. Because of the importance of epidemiology in obesity, it is worth spending some time on examples of how the statistical inference arising from epidemiology stood the test of experimental investigation.

In the 1990s there was a large body of epidemiological evidence, suggesting that our antioxidant status was linked to the risk of cancer and this was supported by cell and experimental studies.[2] Our antioxidant status is based on our habitual intake of certain vitamins and also certain food components that protect our organs from damage by uncontrolled and high levels of free oxygen in cells. Normally, oxygen is carefully transported around the body in specialised delivery systems, the best known of which is hemoglobin. Anxious to put the theory to the test, a consortium of scientists set up a very large study among smokers in China who received various mixtures of antioxidant vitamins or a placebo and were followed for seven years.[3] At the conclusion of the study, no effect of treatment on lung cancer was seen. Many similar studies were completed over the next decade and the vast majority showed no effect. One certainly did and that was conducted by the National Eye Institute, which showed that a particular cocktail of antioxidants reduce the severity of Age Related Macular Degeneration, the main cause of loss of vision in older persons.[4] Other examples of the proof of an epidemiological statistical inference was that between the B vitamin and the risk of the neural tube defect spina bifida[5] or that between the consumption of industrially hardened fats and high levels of blood cholesterol.[6] In some instances, the findings of epidemiological associations between some aspect of diet and disease cannot easily be studied by dietary intervention. But in the vast majority of cases, such associations can be examined using dietary interventions thereby strengthening the policy-making decision process. Regrettably, the body of data on epidemiologically based statistical inference is much greater than that on dietary intervention studies. However, the latter is always the highest level of evidence. Thus throughout this book, the reader needs to appreciate both the value and limitations of epidemiological inferences and obesity, its causes and consequences.

Are You Fat?

The most widely used measure of excessive weight is Body Mass Index (BMI) where one's weight in kilograms is divided by one's height in metres squared (kg/m²). There is a good reason for this. Taller people (adults) are by definition heavier on average than smaller people (children) so, if all we did was to compare groups with different weights we would also be comparing people with different heights. So we adjust weight for height and the method of choice is BMI. As a measure of obesity, it has its strengths and weaknesses and it is worthwhile to spend some time on its origins. These origins began in the apparently most unlikely of places: the US life insurance industry.

In 1912, the Association of Life Insurance Medical Directors issued a report, which documented the contribution of excess weight to mortality from different causes.[7] Their report was based on very extensive actuarial data that the industry routinely gathers to assess risk in life insurance. They defined normal weight as not more than 15% under, or 25% over, the average weight they had observed in their data set. Then in 1942, a statistician at the Metropolitan Life Insurance (MLI) examined data on four million US citizens who had taken out life insurance policies and categorised them into weights for different heights for people with small, medium and large frames.[8] These MLI data were then extensively used to define 'ideal weight'. In 1959, the MLI tables replaced the term 'ideal weight' with 'desirable weight' and in 1983, the tables were simply referred to as weight[9] and height[10] tables. There were recognisable flaws with the MLI data. Firstly, only insured persons were included and in general it could be inferred that the sample was thus biased toward a more healthy and affluent population. Secondly, not all of the data was directly measured as some involved self-reported weight and height and we now know that, on average, people overestimate their height and underestimate their weight. Finally, weights and heights were recorded with subjects wearing full clothing and shoes. Nonetheless, these tables were extensively used in public health to establish 'relative weight', defined as measured body weight divided by the midpoint of medium frame desirable weight. In 1972, the renowned nutritional epidemiologist from the University of Minnesota School of Public Health, Professor Ancel Keys, published a landmark paper, which drew on data on weight and height from the Seven Countries Study.[11] This study was designed primarily to study the links between diet, blood cholesterol and heart disease and was conducted in the US, Italy, Yugoslavia, Japan, Finland, Greece and the Netherlands. They showed that the best indirect measure of fatness was the BMI and, to this day, BMI is the universal basis for deciding adequacy or otherwise of body weight. The exact points on the BMI scale to delineate optimal weight had, however, yet to be established.

In 1985, the US National Institute of Health issued a consensus statement entitled 'The health implications of obesity'.[12] They noted that a BMI corresponding to 20% above ideal weight was equivalent to 27 kg/m^2 based on the

1983 MLI tables and 26kg/m² based on the 1959 tables. They noted that these 1983 BMI values didn't differ radically from the data gathered by the US National Institute of Health statistics of 27.8 for men and 27.3 for women. These US data wouldn't last long. In 1998, the World Health Organization revised these figures downwards based on more globally applicable data to what is used today: normal BMI ranges from 18.99 to 24.99, that of pre-obesity from 25.0 to 29.99 and 30 and above as obese. In the stroke of a pen, millions were re-classified as overweight or obese.[13]

It is thus important to recognise that the definition of obesity (BMI) is based on a correlate of body fatness but is itself not a direct measure of human fatness. One study has examined the relationship between percentage body fat measured using the technique of bioelectrical impedance. Basically bioelectrical impedance operates as follows. A miniscule electric current is run through the body, from one foot on a specialised bathroom scales through the body to the other foot, or from one hand to another in a hand held device. Per unit body weight, the fatter a person is, the less muscle they have. The current runs much faster through the water-rich muscle and thus we get an indirect measure of body fat content. One study has examined the relationship between percentage body fat measured using the technique of bioelectrical impedance and BMI in a large (13,601) sample of US adults.[14] Using a statistical method of evaluating true and false positives, BMI was classed as a 'good' measure of total body fat for men aged less than 60 years and as 'excellent' for women of that age. For those above 60, the true sensitivity was classified as 'fair' for men and again 'excellent' for women. The authors note: 'In our results, BMI showed an un-acceptable low sensitivity for detecting body fatness, with more than half of obese subjects (by body fat measurement) being labeled as normal or over-weight by BMI.' Shorter people are more likely to be deemed overweight on the basis of BMI because of their shorter legs meaning that their trunk, the heaviest part of their body, contributes disproportionately to BMI, compared to taller people.[15]

Notwithstanding the limitations of BMI as a measure of obesity, it is likely to continue to be used to link health outcomes to obesity, simply because it is such an easy set of data to collect. However, there are now excellent hand-held devices that can be used to measure body fat using bioelectrical impedance and which cost less than US $40. These must become part and parcel of all large studies of body weight and health. Alternatives to BMI have been proposed such as waist to hip ratio (WHR). A high WHR implies a bigger belly than hips and is typical of mostly male abdominal obesity. Women tend to have a lower WHR than men giving rise to the gynoid obesity as opposed to male android obesity, also referred to respectively as pear shaped or apple shaped obesity. The process of measuring waist and hip is not nearly as simple as measuring BMI and requires careful training. Moreover, there are different international standards as to how exactly to measure WHR.

The Statistics of Obesity and Health

So measuring obesity is not without its problems and like a lot of population-based nutrition, it is not without its methodological challenges. One such challenge is linking overweight and obesity with health-related issues, of which type 2 diabetes and high blood pressure would be the most significant with both contributing to heart disease. Conventional wisdom is that obesity has a U-shaped nature when plotted against ill health and mortality. That is, there is a central range of BMI values that define a normal weight range and this tends to be flat (BMI range from 25–30). Once you move outside of this range the flat nature disappears. At the lower end, the further you move away from the normal weight range, the higher is the risk of mortality. At the upper end, the further you move away from the normal range, the higher is mortality. Thus BMI values below or above the normal range of BMI 20–5 increase the risk of mortality. That is a universally accepted rule: the obesity–mortality curve is U-shaped, bad to be skinny and bad to be fat. That conventional wisdom hides some challenging facts about the link between mortality and BMI. In 1983, the Royal College of Physicians in London issued a report on obesity in which they examined mortality against BMI in different age groups.[16] Clearly, as we age, mortality rises but the shape of the curve linking mortality from all causes and BMI also changes. The rule that a BMI range of 20–5 is associated with the lowest level of mortality was held true up to the age of 50. For the next decade, mortality rose steadily as BMI fell below 22 and it rose again steadily above a BMI of 30. Thus the optimum range for this age group was 22–30. For those aged 60 to 69 years, the same steady rise in mortality below a BMI of about 22 was again seen but there did not appear to be a rise in obesity above that value. When averaged across all ages, conventional wisdom applied but above the age of 50, this was not the case. Two years later, researchers in the US confirmed that finding and they identified 23 other reports in the literature, which supported the notion that BMI should be looked at differently in different age groups.[17] A more recent paper using quite advanced statistical techniques also showed that as age increases the nadir in the BMI–mortality curve rises from a BMI of about 20 in 20 year olds to about 27 in 70 year olds.[18] Again mortality overall rises with age. Just as importantly as a gradual rise in the nadir of the BMI–mortality curve was the finding that the rise in mortality on either side of this nadir rose considerably. Generally speaking, the normal BMI–mortality curve presented in public health messages is the one for the total population and one can speculate as to why age is generally ignored. First, there is the fear that if the public hears that being a little overweight is not really that bad for health, as we get older, it will diminish the overall message to the population that excess body weight is a bad thing. The second is that research tends to maintain conventional wisdom at all times and given the complete dominance of the total population curve for BMI–mortality links in the literature, in national and international reports and in policy recommendations, fine tuning these curves for different age groups might be seen as a challenge to conventional wisdom. One can sympathise with those in the field of public health in opting for a one-size-fits-all approach to the risks of obesity and the main lesson to be learned from this diminishing impact of obesity on older persons is that all population campaigns that target weight management should have children, adolescents and younger adults as their priority audience. Nonetheless, health professionals must also adopt a slightly more forgiving attitude to their advice to older persons with respect to body weight.

BMI and Mortality: Confronting New Challenges

Challenges to conventional wisdom may be rare, but they do occur and a distinguished epidemiologist at the US National Center for Health Statistics, Dr Katherine Flegal led such a challenge with a paper published in 2012.[19] In 2013, her team took a look at the global literature and ended up examining data from 97 studies, involving 2.88 million people with 270,000 deaths. The same pattern was found. The nadir in the BMI–mortality link was found in what is deemed by conventional wisdom to be overweight with a BMI of 25–30. Of course, this did not go down with some people and especially so at the Harvard School of Public Health where a conference was quickly organised to explain the errors in Dr Flegal's work. The furore reached to the dizzy levels of *Nature*, perhaps the most prestigious scientific journal around.[20] One world-renowned Harvard don was reported to have stated that: 'This study [Flegal's] is really a pile of rubbish, and no one should waste their time reading it.' The *Nature* article tried to make sense of the differences pointing out that big epidemiological data analysis is complex and sorting out confounding factors is not easy. The Harvard group argues that the rise in obesity at lower BMI values is associated with smokers who tend to be thin and at higher risk of death and also by people who are sick or ill and who are again thin as a result and also with a higher risk of mortality. So, in one large study, they examined the BMI–mortality link having removed smokers and those who died within four years of the start of the study.[21] Now they found a linear relationship between BMI and mortality. Flegal, on the other hand, argues that removing smokers or ex-smokers creates a possible bias toward a better-educated and healthier population. She also argues that the Harvard studies rely on self-reported weight and height and, generally speaking, people on average under-report their weight and over-report their height. The argument may go on but more and more data are emerging showing that people who are overweight but not obese survive some of the obesity-related illnesses better than those who are slim. Quite why we don't know but some have suggested that having spare energy stores as fat may become important in certain instances involving disease onset. Does this mean that the time has come to abandon the conventionally accepted optimal range for BMI? My answer is not to do so. Firstly, we need to be careful to distinguish between the development of a disease (morbidity) and death from that disease (mortality). The latter is easier to measure for epidemiologists who can access official death certificates. However, in studying morbidity (disease) rates, confirmation of the diagnosis of a disease through a questionnaire begs the question as to the reliability of the diagnosis. An individual may report having been diagnosed with high blood pressure by a health professional but that might be less than 100% trustworthy. Who diagnosed the condition? How was it diagnosed? What cut-off point or reference standard for blood pressure was used? These are important questions if an epidemiological study is to be the basis of making a policy decision. So for now, it is certainly best to retain the existing values for BMI used to categorise people into different grades of body weight. However, the discipline of epidemiology must resolve the current debate on the apparently conflicting interpretations of the optimal BMI range. That does not mean that one side of the debate 'wins'. It means that society gets what it is entitled to, namely the best advice on diet, health and obesity.

The Challenges of Using Large Dietary Survey Data

Truth is actually a hard thing to find when it comes to the next phase of studying obesity. We have seen that BMI is not quite like the boiling point of water in its exactitude. We have seen that the link between BMI and mortality is not quite as clear-cut as it is made out to be. Next we move to the dietary dimension of food, body weight and health, and here we find yet another challenge to the data. There are many techniques available to measure food intake and for the purposes of this book, it serves little value to describe these in detail. Some require people to recall past eating events while others require people to actively record actual eating events. Either way, the nutritional epidemiologist ends up with two key sets of data: average daily intake of foods and average daily intake of nutrients. So now we can divide our population into groups of body weight from low to high and examine the patterns of food and nutrient intake across extremes of body weight. But there is a problem.

It has long been known that such surveys lead to an underestimate of food intake.[22] First let me present my personal theory as to how this can be explained. Most people in today's world struggle with their weight and many seek to downsize through dieting. Usually, dieting starts on a Monday. All goes well with the diet but come Thursday any little excitement or disappointment can derail the process and the diet ends and normal food intake returns. When we ask people to take part in a dietary survey, we stress that they must honestly report their true food intake. Now the subject has a choice. Is the Monday to Wednesday healthy eating the true norm or is the Thursday to Sunday standard unrestricted food intake the true norm? They may choose the former or a mixture of the two. Either way, a large number of participants report intakes of calories and nutrients that are biologically implausible. We know this through the use of what are called independent biomarkers.

For example, we can ask volunteers to collect all their urine for 24 hours and measure the quantity of nitrogen excreted over that single day. We convert nitrogen back to protein equivalents so we know exactly how much protein was consumed that day.[23] The reported intake of protein should exactly equal the quantity estimated from urine. It doesn't in a large number of cases. We can also use many other sophisticated methods to obtain independent data on the intake of such nutrients as energy, salt or protein. All of these techniques show that energy under-reporting is widespread, affecting as many as 20–60% of subjects. Older persons, females and most importantly overweight and obese persons are most likely to under-report.

Epidemiologists have long used various techniques to adjust for energy under-reporting and such techniques often rely on an assumption that the intake of a given nutrient correlates highly with the intakes of calories. That must be true for those nutrients that actually contribute to caloric intake such as carbohydrate, fat and protein. These nutrients are widespread in the human food chain. But nutrients such as zinc or calcium, vitamin C or fibre, tend to have a very narrow food base and thus it is difficult, or to this writer impossible, to see how fancy statistical gymnastics of modern epidemiology can correct the intakes of these nutrients for under-reporting. Under-reporting of foods presents an even greater challenge. Epidemiologists might be able to link reported nutrient intake with reported energy intake since all humans must eat all nutrients or eventually become sick and ultimately die. That is not so with foods. Some people never eat eggs or prawns or cows' milk or coffee or alcohol or mustard or Chinese food or whatever. How can such non-consumers ever be included in data correction based on reported caloric intake? Thus whereas the data linking nutrient intake and obesity has its flaws, that of food intake and obesity is utterly doomed. The future may involve advanced biomarkers using very modern analytical methods that draw simultaneously on the presence of hundreds of metabolites in blood and urine and employ pattern recognition techniques to try to find patterns of metabolites that correspond with particular nutrient profiles.[24] It is however, a science presently in its infancy and many doubt that biomarkers are the panacea that some would make them out to be.

In basic biology, it is possible to reduce all confounding factors and study just one element in complete laboratory isolation. It might be a single enzyme or a cell or an isolated organ or an inbred mouse living under very strict experimental conditions. That's easy. Studying human behaviour at population level is inordinately more challenging. Obesity remains a serious global health problem that is linked both to changing energy intake and to changing physical activity patterns. In this chapter we have seen that our main measure of body fat, BMI, is imperfect. We have seen that there are important questions to ask of the links between BMI and mortality rates. That doesn't mean that we relent in any way in reducing the burden of human suffering from excess weight. But it does bode nutrition research to rethink and constantly strive to improve its methodology. So, we have come to define obesity and its risks and the issue of measuring nutrient and food intake. Flaws abound in all but this writer is conservative and believes that we must live with what we have, albeit constantly improving such tools. Now that we have a handle on the tools for measuring obesity, we need to turn to the scale of the problem of overweight and obesity.

CHAPTER THREE

Human Obesity: Old and New

In his best-selling book *The End of Overeating* David Kessler wrote thus:

> For thousands of years human body weight stayed remarkably stable. Throughout adulthood we basically consumed no more than the food we needed to burn. People who were overweight stood apart from the general population. Millions of calories passed through our bodies, yet with rare exception our weight neither rose nor fell by any significant amount. A perfect biological system seemed to be at work. Then in the 1980s something changed.[1]

What was deemed to have changed was an epidemic of obesity with one third of the US population overweight. If the prevalence of obesity was held to have started in the 1980s then, rightly, Kessler could argue that the causes of that epidemic were also temporal. Some aspect of the food chain and some features of lifestyle had changed such that they created the conditions, which allowed this epidemic to blossom. But what if Kessler is wrong? What if we were to find records of obesity and overweight that show the problem existed throughout history? Quite simply, it would mean that the causes of obesity are not as clear-cut as would be assumed if the whole problem took off in the 1980s. I intend to show that, indeed, Kessler is wrong. Obesity has always been with us wherever and whenever we prospered and moreover the modern epidemic of obesity began in the nineteenth century, not the 1980s.

In 2008, researchers at the University of Tübingen discovered a female figurine that was produced as long ago as 35,000 years during the upper Palaeolithic period.[2] Measuring just six centimetres (2.4 inches) it depicts a grossly obese female, with large pendulous breasts, severe abdominal obesity and fat thighs and arms. Such figurines depicting Venus have been found in many locations and across many millennia. Venus of Dolní V stonice is dated as 29,000 years old and the Venus of Willendorf is about 25,000 years old.

These obese figurines, which emphasise the female sexual form, are believed to be devoted to female reproductive capacity. One expert in the field commented in 1939 that: 'The women immortalized in Stone Age sculpture were fat; there is no other word for it. Obesity was already a fact of life for palaeolithic man – at least for palaeolithic women.'[3]

Obesity in the Graeco-Roman Era

Moving onward in time to several centuries BC, we can read the opinions of the famous Greek physicians and draw on the excellent historic reviews of David Haslam.[4] In *On Airs, Waters, Places*, the earliest text on public health, Hippocrates documents childhood obesity among the Scythian race (in modern Iran) as follows:

> The male children, until they are old enough to ride, spend most of their time sitting in the wagons and they walk very little since they are so often changing their place of residence. The girls get amazingly flabby and podgy.

He quotes many other Greek and Egyptian physicians and philosophers on obesity, its cause and cures. Herodotus wrote: 'Egyptians vomit and purge themselves thrice every month, with a view to preserve their health, which in their opinion is chiefly injured by their aliment.' Pythagoras is quoted as saying that: 'No man, who values his health, ought to trespass on the bounds of moderation, either in labour, diet or concubinage.'

Haslam cites Hippocrates rightly predicting the balance between energy in and energy out:

> It is very injurious to health to take in more food than the constitution will bear, when, at the same time one uses no exercises to carry off the excess. For as aliment fills, and exercise empties the body, the result of an exact equipoise between them must be to leave the body in the same state they found it, that is, in perfect health.

A non-physician, Plutarch made the point that: 'Thin people are generally the most healthy; we should therefore not indulge our appetites with delicacies or high living, for fear of growing corpulent.'

It is abundantly clear that the overweight and obese were a feature of ancient Greece, which it must be remembered, fostered great affluence and the advent of new foods from the far flung corners of its empire. Whereas these citations dismiss the point made by Kessler that 'A perfect biological system seemed to work', they don't yet quantify the extent of obesity. Now let us turn to some historical data of opinion on the prevalence of obesity and later we will move from opinion to fact as we approach the nineteenth century. The Roman agronomist Lucius Columella (65AD) writing in his famous text *De Re Rustica* commented as follows on Roman youth: 'The consequence is that ill health attends so slothful a manner of living; for the bodies of our young men are so flabby and enervated that death seems likely to make no change to them.'[5]

Obesity in the Renaissance Era

Moving forward in time to the wealthy city of Venice, we encounter the remarkable Luigi Cornaro (1550 AD) who, in his mid-80s wrote a book on longevity *The Art of Living Long.*[6] He first comments on the failings of life in Italy: 'It is in consequence force of habit, that of late, indeed during my own lifetime and memory, three evil customs have gradually gained a foothold in our own Italy. The first of these is adulation and ceremony. The second is heresy and the third is intemperance.' He then goes on to say: 'Coming, then, to that evil concerning which I propose to speak, – the vice of intemperance, – I declare that it is a wicked thing that it should prevail to such an extent as to greatly lower, nay almost abolish, the temperate life.'

Here Cornaro is describing not an isolated lifestyle of over indulgence but a pandemic rate of poor nutrition. He then goes on to provide a vivid description of how prevalent obesity was in the Italy of his day:

> O wretched and unhappy Italy, canst thou not see that intemperance kills every year amongst thy people as great a number as would perish during the time of a most dreadful pestilence, or by the sword or fire of many bloody wars. And these truly immoral banquets of thine, now so commonly the custom, – feasts so great and intolerable that the tables found are never large enough to accommodate the innumerable dishes set upon them, so that they may be heaped, one upon another, almost mountain high, – must we not brand them with so many destructive battles. Who could ever live amid such a multitude of disorders and excessed. Oh for the love of God, I conjure you to apply a remedy to this unholy condition.

It is very clear from this that overeating and obesity was leading to widespread premature death in Venice at this time and no doubt in Rome, Florence and all the other wealthy cities of Italy. Again, it challenges Kessler's concept that all was hunky-dory until the mid-twentieth century. To describe the death rate from obesity as likening that of 'dreadful pestilence' or 'the sword or fire of many bloody wars' is to state that obesity is an epidemic of grave public health proportions.

Obesity in the Age of Enlightenment

In the mid-eighteenth century, at the funeral of the famed obese Daniel Lambert, who had an extraordinary Body Mass Index of 132 kg/m² (30–5 is obese!), the distinguished physician, Thomas Short was reported to have said: 'I believe no Age did ever afford more instances of corpulency than our own.'[7] Just a few years after Lambert died in 1806, Sir William Wadd wrote in his famous book, *Cursory Remarks on Corpulence*, in 1816: 'If the increase of wealth and the refinement of modern times, have tended to banish plague and pestilence from our cities, they have probably introduced the increased frequency of corpulence. For every 1 fat person in Spain or France, there are 100 in England.'[8]

For the first time Sir William also raises the issue of the built environment and its role in obesity. He cites the *Holingshed's Chronicles*, a collaborative series of two volumes published in 1577 and 1587. Wadd writes thus:

> Hollingshed who lived in Queen Elizabeth's reign, speaking of the increase of luxury in his days notices, 'the multitude of chimneys erected lately; whereas in the sound remembrance of some old men, there were not two or three, if so many, in most uplandish towns of the realm.'

Tongue in cheek, Wadd then writes: 'How far corpulency has kept pace with the numbers of chimnies, I prefer not to determine.'

So far we have seen no evidence of obesity as rare such that 'People who were overweight were a rare event', as Kessler affirmed. Wadd in his book cited above in 1816 does raise the issue of social class:

> For it must be admitted that the lower orders of society, the poor and the laborious are seldom thus encumbered and it is only among those who have the

means of obtaining the comforts of life, without labour, that excessive corpulency is met with. You may see an army of forty thousand foot soldiers without a fat man. And I affirm, that by plenty, and rest twenty of the forty will grow fat.

Obesity in the New Industrial Era

In 1908, Dr Brandreth Symonds, MD, chief medical officer of the Mutual Life Insurance Company of New York presented a paper to the Medical Society of New Jersey entitled 'The influence of overweight and underweight on vitality'.[9] It was to be the very first paper directly linking weight and, in particular, excess weight to health and the data he used was gathered from 1889 onwards by the Association of Life Insurance Medical Directors of America and the Actuarial Society of America. Symonds showed that compared to 'underweights', those who were 'overweights' were six times more likely to develop diabetes, twice as likely to develop stroke and 50% more likely to develop heart disease. Symonds worked on weight and mortality relationships in men aged 15 to 69 so if we assume that the data were gathered around 1895, then he included men born in the 1820s, some 40 years before the American Civil War. These data show that contrary to what we are led to believe is a modern epidemic we had obesity linked to health well over a century ago.

There are other sources of data, which support this historical analysis and they rely on the use of birth cohorts and the value of birth cohort data to obesity is worth elaborating. If a national survey of weight and height is completed, the data refer only to the date of measurement. They cannot tell us when an individual might have become overweight or obese, given that the sample will be comprised of individuals ranging in age from teens to 90s. One person might have been fat for decades, another might have gained weight only recently while another might have been overweight but recently lost it. Similarly, if a sample was taken in 1960, the extent to which subjects watched television would vary very considerably. A 60-year-old subject would have spent half their life in a television free environment. However, if a birth cohort born in 1960 is followed thereafter, then they all experience the same opportunity for television viewing and they all have the same experience of world events and technological advances. The US National Bureau of Economic Research has examined the birth cohort changes in BMI using data collected by the National Center for Health Statistics covering subjects born between 1882 and 1986.[10] Its results show that in 1880, average BMI was within the normal weight range (20–5 kg/m^2) at about 22.

Mean BMI of black females reached 25 by 1900, while for white males, black males and white females, the dates that a mean BMI of 25 was achieved were, respectively, 1905, 1915 and 1920. Again black females led the way in achieving a BMI in excess of 30 by the year 1940 with all others achieving this by about 1960. Another set of research from the same US Bureau provides data on the BMI of US military recruits from 1864 to 1991. These are more robust data because they are based not on statistical models but on directly measured weight and height. If we take men aged 45 years, the average BMI increased from 23.3 to 26.5 over this time period but the greatest part of this increase (60%) was in the period 1894 to 1961. Only 20% of the rise in BMI was explained post 1961.[11]

We can also look at more modern data gathered in Denmark and which looks at the rate of change in body weight in two groups.[12] The first are 19-year-old military recruits studied since 1945. The second is a set of children aged seven, eight, nine, ten and eleven years, all born in 1930. In both cases, the prevalence of obesity was low at the outset of the studies at about three obese persons per thousand of the population. That trebled by 1960 but, remarkably, it did not change at all between 1960 and 1990. However thereafter obesity again trebled to a level of about 30–40 obese persons per 1,000 of the population. This wave-like growth in obesity, which I call the tsunami of lard, has also been recorded by the researchers at the US Bureau of Economic Research in their 1882–1991 modelling of the growth of obesity in the US.

Obesity and Life Expectance among Today's Children

It is thus clear that overweight and obesity have been with mankind ever since excess food was available to society, where sections of society were affluent enough to be able to afford ample supply of food and when wealth allowed for the evolution of a sedentary lifestyle. It did not all happen in the 1980s as David Kessler implies. For certain, there has been a dramatic rise across the globes with the plague of excess weight now reaching to every corner of the globe. It is also the case that the number of overweight and obese persons has soared in the developed world, particularly at the extremes of excess weight. The World Health Organization regards excess body weight as one of its greatest public health challenges. All of this has led to considerable fears for future generations with statements such as 'This may be the first generation where children will have lower life expectancy than their parents, leaving a huge social gap in family relationships and caring for older family members' from the Irish National

Task Force on Obesity,[13] or 'Because of the increasing rates of obesity, un-healthy eating habits, and physical inactivity, we may see the first generation that will be less healthy and have a shorter life expectancy than their parents' from the US Surgeon General.[14] In general, many of the reviews and reports on the future of the obesity epidemic predict similar dire consequences for this generation. However, in more recent times, several scientific papers have emerged to show that the fears expressed above about parents outliving their obese children may not be realistic. One important paper reviewed the data from nine countries (Australia, China, England, France, Netherlands, New Zealand, Sweden, Switzerland and USA).[15] There are too much data in the paper to delve into in this chapter so let's consider the findings from two countries. Of the obesity rates in Australia, the authors show that: 'The estimated prevalence of overweight including obesity in boys rose from 10% in 1985, to 22% in 1996, to 24% in 2008. In girls, the estimated prevalence rose from 12% in 1985, to 24% in 1996, to 25% in 2008.' These conclusions were based on 41 surveys of childhood weight status conducted between 1985 and 2008 and included data on 264,905 Australians aged 2–18 years. In contrast to Australia where obesity rates are high, the Netherlands has consistently shown low rates of obesity. Their data show that:

In Dutch girls, a 14% decline in overweight including obesity was found from 1999 to 2007. Data for Dutch boys showed a similar significant decrease in 3 – 6-year-olds. Surinamese South Asian (15.0%) and Moroccan (23.0%) children, and Dutch boys (11.3%) showed an overall stabilization of overweight including obesity prevalence between 1999 and 2007. There was however a strong and significant increase in overweight including obesity prevalence in Turkish boys, from 22.4% (1999) to 34.5% (2007), and in Turkish girls, from 27.4–33.8%.

The emerging evidence that obesity rates might be stabilising led the US National Center for Health Statistics to examine available data in the US over the period 2003–4 to 2011–12 reaching the conclusion that:

Among infants and toddlers from birth to aged 2 years, there was no significant change in high weight-for-length prevalence. Among children and adolescents aged 2 to 19 years, there was no significant change overall but there was a significant decrease in obesity prevalence among 2- to 5-year-old children. Among adults, there was no significant change in obesity prevalence in the total population but there was an increase in prevalence among adults aged 60 years and older.[16]

Naturally, when the predicted tidal wave of future obesity levels appeared not to be happening, scientists became nervous and wondered whether this stabilisation was really true or a simple error in survey methods, confounded by some unknown factors. The Prevention and Public Health Task Force of the European Association for the Study of Obesity set out to consider all possible explanations for the observation of a global stabilisation in the rates of obesity.[17] For example, is it the case that as more and more people become obese, their participation in surveys declines and thus the true incidence is underestimated? Is there a publication bias in that scientists are not necessarily reporting higher rates of obesity because that is old news whereas a decile or stabilisation of obesity rates is a hot topic? Is it possible that we are aggregating the data such that in some groups obesity is falling while in others it is rising, yielding a net zero growth? The authors considered these and many other factors and reached the conclusion that: 'On the whole however, the available trend data seem to stand up to scrutiny concerning the most plausible biases and interpretational errors.'

One of the most popular explanations of this stabilisation is that the obesogenic environment we live in has now claimed all the genetically sensitive individuals, an issue we will explore in depth later. That is an attractive argument if the growth of obesity is seen as linear, steadily rising year after year. But, as I have shown in this chapter, that is not how the epidemic of obesity has occurred. The growth in obesity has been wave-like, rising, stabilising and then rising again. Thus there is no room for complacency. Obesity is a major global public health problem that will cost the taxpayer a mighty chunk of their health care spend. Stabilisation in the rise of obesity does not mean that obesity is conquered. However, this chapter has shown that obesity has always been with us and that the modern epidemic of obesity did not start in the 1980s. Maybe we are really seeing the advent stabilisation of the growth of obesity among some groups in a limited number of developed economies. However, as is repeatedly argued throughout this book, unless governments invest proportionately in obesity prevention, these successes may simply be sporadic and may fail to meet the true potential to tackle the modern plague of obesity. Just as the common belief is that obesity is a truly modern phenomenon, an equally strongly held belief is that this modern epidemic is due to the advent of modern food processing. It is to that issue that we now turn.

CHAPTER FOUR

The Human Food Chain: Old and New

It is almost a given that when obesity is mentioned in the media today, it will be accompanied by the term 'processed foods'. Indeed to emphasise the matter further, some researchers are now choosing to use the term 'ultra-processed foods'. Either way the message is clear: the modern obesity epidemic is directly linked to the food industry that peddles these processed or ultra-processed foods. The implications are two-fold: the first is that processed foods have become such a mainstream of today's diet that we are passively overeating on foods laced with hidden fats, sugars and salt. The second is that the advent of processed and ultra-processed foods is a new phenomenon largely developed in the last half century. The following quotes serve to illustrate how popular books, social media and scientific advocates associate modern food processing with the obesity epidemic and with a food industry determined to sell us more of their food in a highly competitive market:

> It's true that foods have long been processed in order to preserve them, as when we pickle or ferment or smoke, but industrial processing aims to do much more than extend shelf life. Today foods are processed in ways specifically designed to sell us more food by pushing our evolutionary buttons – our inborn prefer-ences for sweetness and fat and salt. These qualities are difficult to find in nature but cheap and easy for the food scientist to deploy, with the result that processing induces us to consume much more of these ecological rarities than is good for us. (Michael Pollan in his book *In Defence of Food*)[1]

> The rapid rise in consumption of ultra-processed food and drink products, especially since the 1980s, is the main dietary cause of the concurrent rapid rise in obesity and related diseases throughout the world. (Marion Nestlé, author and academic writing in *The Atlantic* quoting Professor Carlos Monteiro of the University of São Paulo)[2]

Until the food industry, the grocery industry, and the restaurant industry realize that it is not in their best interest to provide our current food choices, don't expect our global food environment to improve anytime soon. (Dr Robert Lustig in his book *Fat Chance*)[3]

These quotations speak for themselves as to how many influential writers and academics view processed foods. I will return to these later in this chapter but not until I have had the chance to outline the major milestones, which over time have cumulatively shaped the modern food supply. Of these, I have selected six to illustrate this development. As in the previous chapter, which outlined the evolution of obesity, a look back in time is central to understanding why we are where we are today. As Mark Twain said, 'History doesn't repeat itself but it rhymes.'

Milestone #1: Fire

In his book *Catching Fire: How Cooking Made Us Human*, Richard Wrangham describes how the control of fire and the advent of cooked meals represented one of the greatest transitions in the evolution of man.[4] Initially, fire was the outcome of an accident such as bush fires that we regularly see today on television news across the globe. Lightening, intense heat, dryness, gaseous emissions from the volatile oils of trees such as eucalyptus and accidents such as sparks flying from an intended or unintended clash of stones, all contributed to the outbreak of fire. Wrangham imagines some young men at the conclusion of such a fire swirling the dying embers of branches through the air and marvelling at the process of re-ignition. Somehow, the advantages of such accidental fire on the palatability of foods caught the imagination of early hominids and, in time, they learned ways of creating and conserving their own fires. One of the big effects of cooking was that the biologically available calories from food dramatically increased. There are many studies available to show that rats perform far better in terms of normal growth when fed cooked vegetable foods such as potatoes or cooked meats such as beef when compared to the raw form of these foods. However, Professor Claus Leitzmann reported one of the most revealing studies on the biological effects of raw foods from the University of Giessen in Germany.[5] His group studied female 'raw foodists', aged less than 45 years who were not pregnant and who consumed raw foods to varying degrees. As the level of foods consumed in the raw form rose from 70 to 100% of all food intake, average body mass index fell from 21.2 to 19.3 kg/m². In other words these women who were adherers to a raw diet went from thin to dangerously skinny as the level of raw food in the diet rose. Interestingly, the proportion of women with amenorrhea, a failure to menstruate, rose from 10% among the group with the lowest intake of raw foods to almost 50% among those exclusively devoted to the consumption of raw foods. This paper illustrates how raw foods reduce the amount of energy available from foodstuffs. Data from the US among vegetarians show that those who cooked their food had an average BMI of 24 compared to vegetarians who ate only raw foods whose mean BMI was 20.4.[6]

Anthropologists have calculated the average distances travelled daily in search of foods by human foragers among the !kung and Ache civilisations compared to chimpanzees. The human foragers travelled 10–20 km/d expending 40% of total calories on this exercise. In contrast, chimpanzees travelled a mere 3–5 km/d, which consumed 29% of their calories. Thus the evolutionary advantage to those who had access to cooked as well as to raw food was enormous and as a result, evolution adapted human physiology to favour those eating cooked foods. In humans anatomical adaptations that favoured cooked foods began in the mouth, which compared to other animals is quite small with fewer molars (the teeth at the back of the mouth used for grinding foods), and this was associated with thinner jaw-bones and smaller chewing muscles. In addition, our hindgut shrank dramatically since we relied less on gut bacteria to extract calories from fibrous vegetable matter. Our more efficient anatomy coupled with an ability to extract the maximum nutrients from foods meant that more energy was available for those who were genetically capable of developing larger brains. The human brain is like any great supercomputer and demands an enormous amount of energy, in return generating very large quantities of heat. A newborn baby uses 75% of its energy for post-natal brain development as all the wires are urgently connected so that the child can learn its language, music, culture, gastronomy, etiquette, manners and so forth.[7] This falls to 59% at four years but in adulthood, it stays constant at about 25% of total caloric intake. For most westerners living a sedentary life, the brain consumes twice as much energy as everyday volitional exercise. Bigger brains meant a greater capacity for more complex thinking such as the utilisation of fire for cooking.

Milestone #2: Cooking

One can imagine early man exploring the debris after a wild fire and discovering the scarred body of a dead pig, suitably cooked in the glowing embers of the fading fire. Not to pass up on a meal, the inquisitive man or woman might have let it cool and then butchered it as normal only to discover the wonders of pork crackling and roast pork. There was no going back for that community. As soon as fire was captured and managed, one can envisage some crude spit used to cook a whole animal or, in the case of larger animals, sticks would have been used to hang lumps of raw meat over the heat of the fire until cooked to taste. In time, the capacity of heated stones on which to cook would have emerged and then there would have been the advent of pit cooking where a hole in the ground was layered with heated stones and food cooked in a semi sealed environment. Then boiling water would have served to transfer the heat from the fire to a more manageable mode of cooking.

As with all innovation in the human food chain, to focus on the scientific or technical aspect alone is to miss the really significant outcome. In the case of fire and the advent of cooking there were several profoundly important consequences to society. Firstly, cooking killed food-borne parasites such as worms and killed potentially dangerous bacteria. Cooked meat could then be kept without putre-faction if the storage conditions were cool and dry and early man would have discovered this. Cooking would also have destroyed natural toxins in plants, which abound in many raw foods causing a loss of nutritional value or, indeed, a wide variety of illnesses such as neurotoxins in green potatoes, gut toxins in uncooked beans or hallucinatory compounds in certain raw mushrooms. But it was the social impact of fire and cooking which made the most profound impact on human development. Hunting, killing, transporting prey, skinning, butchering, tending fires, making spearheads, spear shafts and flints for starting fires, cooking, drying hides and so forth all required one truly amazing human achievement: the division of labour. We are the only species that entrusts the procurement of our food supply to others: 'I'll make you a very sharp and strong spear if you give me some of the animal you kill with it!' No other species does this. A second social outcome of fire and cooking was the advent of cave dwelling. A fire on the open plains has three big disadvantages. Firstly, it can attract the interests of other communities passing by, some of whom might not be so friendly. Secondly, in the chill of the night and the cold of the winter, a fire in the open is hugely inefficient save for the lucky few who can huddle nearby. Finally, heavy rain can wipe out a fire. Within the cave, the community had privacy from unwelcome guests, they had a very efficient capture of heat and the rains were no threat. Two other great adjustments to human life ensued.

If you ever watch a colony of primates sitting around the forest, you will see it spend hours preening one another, literally picking off parasites such as lice and the like. Such skin or ecto-parasites can cause great suffering and are highly contagious so it is in everyone's interest to invest in this communal 'public health' activity – 'You scratch my back and I'll scratch yours' approach. With fire and controlled heat, a new selective evolutionary pressure point arose. Those with fewer hairs could warm themselves within the cave and not be too bothered about ecto-parasites. Soon the 'naked ape' emerged with no hair.[8] However, to wander out to hunt at night or to travel long distances with poor weather required the naked ape to adopt to clothing for warmth and so the hides of hunted animals were treated and then worked into wearable, water-proof and warm garments allowing man to forage further upland where fewer competitors would be found and where they would have the advantage of a more abundant food chain. The division of labour meant that these warriors and adventurers didn't have to worry about the provisions for such excursions; they now had tailors, tanners and cobblers to provide them with the best of clothing. The big civilising impact of fire and cooking was the development of increasingly civilised societies. The morality of group existence developed to a new level. Language evolved with eventually music of sorts and painting and storytelling and the building of deep communal ties. The tiresome days of living on the plains chasing dangerous animals with crude weapons, encoun-tering unwelcome strangers, exposed to the elements and expending vast amounts of energy just to stay alive, were gone. Man had a firm foothold on civilisation, which no other species would ever enjoy. 'Go hither fox. This is man-space!'

Milestone #3: Farming

Whereas caves were a great solution to the early challenges of community living, they quickly became outdated. The safety of caves meant that family life was less arduous than out on the Svelte but soon population expansion meant that caves had to be abandoned. However, by now, many generations had learned the morals and ethics of a semi-civilised society. They were brighter, better equipped, more ambitious, more organised and with a greater control of communication than their forebears who first entered cave dwellings. They had unity of purpose and common gossip, myths and early religions to bind them into strong social units. Some would have settled near the fertile deltas of rivers giving themselves access to prey, which was easy and non-threatening to hunt such as birds of flight, fish and waterfowl.[9] They then had access to eggs and shellfish, all of which were rich in the types of fatty acids, which the brain specifically requires. Oyster 'middens' or mounds of oyster shells are a worldwide phenomenon and a great example are the Whaleback middens along opposite sides of the banks of the Damariscotta River in Maine. The volume has been estimated at a staggering 45 million cubic feet.[10]

But to move from hunting to farming was yet another step. We tend to think of herds of wild buffalo and the like when we envisage the challenges of the first introduction of domesticated animal husbandry. However, as Felipe Fernández-Armesto points out in his excellent book *Food: A History*, the earliest successes in animal husbandry were in snail farming.[11] In putting forward this concept he writes in its favour thus: 'Snail farming is so simple, so technically undemanding and so close conceptually to the habitual food garnering methods of gatherers that it seems pig-headedly doctrinaire to exclude the possibility.' The Franchthi Caves that lie along the Aegean Sea of the Greek Peloponnese are famed for their huge deposits of snail shells dating back to 10,700 BC. Fernández-Armesto points out that, 4,000 years later, the snail shell mounds were augmented in turn by mounds of red deer bones and the bones of tuna fish.

However, at some stage, the domestication of large animals occurred and it has been suggested that the transition started when man began to develop a symbiotic relationship with herds of cattle. The herds were managed in their drifting toward the best and freshest pastures using a variety of techniques one of which was fire. Over time, the cattle and the herders developed a mutual respect. But herding isn't farming so my guess is simply that young bull and cow calves were taken from the herd and managed in settlements. The animals were bred and calves would have been carefully selected from the herd on the basis of desirable paternal or maternal qualities. It would take no more than a few generations for such domesticated animals to become docile and adapted to the animal husbandry techniques of the day, including of course the milking of dairy cows. Milk would have been highly valued as a food and quite likely, it was the nourishment from milk that tipped the scales from herding to farming. Dairying is difficult to manage in drifting herds and to be really worthwhile, requires domestication with the establishment of the necessary infrastructure for the collection and processing of milk, which also supplies butter, cheese, yogurt and cream. Bull calves can be reared for slaughter ensuring an adequate supply of meat as well as hides for clothes and horns for musical instruments. And so the time came to settle down and become the very first dairy farmers.

It is quite a different matter for the domestication of agricultural crops. As Fernández-Armesto points out, the gatherer had become very sophisticated in the art of foraging. No longer was it hit-and-miss. Now a wealth of knowledge had been built up and passed on through generations as to where to go for the best crops, fruit, berries, tubers and the like. To quote the great agronomist Jack Harlan: 'Gatherers understand the life cycles of plants, know the seasons of the year, and when and where the natural plant resources can be harvested in great abundance with the least effort.'[12]

If the gatherers were so advanced in their ways, which, according to Fernández-Armesto included sowing seeds, using fire to clear areas for re-growth and the establishment of private land rights, why would the domestication of crops be so attractive, such that in time and up to the present date mankind is dependent on crop husbandry for all its plant food and all its animal food reared on plants? A wide range of options has been put forward by Fernández-Armesto as to why crop husbandry evolved including an adaptation to climate change or population growth, a growing food crisis, or societal pressure, or religion. Only a few of these stand up to scrutiny. Population expansion meant that the efficiency of farmed food would ultimately outweigh that of foraging. In his classic article, 'The worst mistake in the history of man', Jared Diamond wrote as follows to explain why our hunter-gatherer ancestors embraced agriculture:

> Of course they adopted it because agriculture is an efficient way to get more food for less work. Planted crops yield far more tons per acre than roots and berries. Just imagine a band of savages, exhausted from searching for nuts or chasing wild animals, suddenly gazing for the first time at a fruit laden orchard or a pasture full of sheep. How many milliseconds do you think it would take them to appreciate the advantages of agriculture?[13]

If population expansion was the tipping point to an agricultural way of life, power and wealth were to sustain it through thick and thin throughout many centuries. Some leaders saw the limitations of foraging and they began to dream of extending those little patches they planted in the fire scorched earth to larger fields to yield food, which not only served to feed the community but which also allowed a substantial surplus to be stored. Such a surplus would have two benefits. Surplus crops could be traded for luxuries with passing traders and could be used to feed small armies to take what wasn't theirs. For sure, these leaders would not be the ones to plough up the land, sow seeds, manage weeds and harvest crops. This was no hippy commune. For just as there were strong leaders, who acquired land as their private wealth, there were serfs who would work this land in kind and foul weather. Early agriculture was cruel and remained so right through history, up to slavery and beyond and, indeed, up to the advent of farm mechanisation. Researchers have compared the health of hunter-gatherers with those of the new agricultural era.[14] Height fell by six inches from the five foot nine inches of the hunter-gatherer male. Life expectancy fell from 26 to 19 years. Diseases such as anaemia increased four-fold and those of bone increased three-fold. The population density of the farming communities was 100 times greater than that among hunter-gatherers such that parasitic infestations and both respiratory and gastrointestinal infections increased. Settled agricultural communities were also subject to hunger and famine if their main or only crop failed for climatic or biological reasons. So why was this agricultural revolution so successful that it dominated all food chains for all times? The simple answer was that it was an efficient system that generated surpluses, which met the needs of ruthless leaders whose average height and life expectancy certainly did not fall. Tribalism abounded and capitalism ruled. Animal and crop husbandry were here to stay and with it all the social inequalities that has haunted man since the idyllic but doomed days of the hunter-gatherer. We presently live in an era where many of the worried well in society have a romantic view of agriculture. It was never romantic. As Jared Diamond wrote:

> Besides malnutrition, starvation and epidemic diseases, farming helped bring another curse upon humanity: deep class divisions. Hunter-gatherers have little or no stored foods and no concentrated food sources, like an orchard or a herd of cows: they live off wild plants and animals they obtain each day. Therefore there can be no kings, no social parasites who grew fat on food seized from others. Only in a farming population could a healthy, non-producing elite set itself above the disease-ridden masses.[15]

Maybe the biblical prediction of the consequences of exiting the luxurious Garden of Eden has a ring of truth or irony: 'I have placed a curse on the ground.

All your life you will struggle to scratch a living from it. It will grow thorns and thistles for you though you will eat its grains. All your life you will sweat to produce food, until your dying day.'[16]

Milestone #4: Innovation and Transformation

One of the explanations put forward for the development of agriculture was the theory that new tools and technologies were invented, which fostered the growth of agriculture. Anthropologists have generally dismissed this in favour of the 'demand' theory arising for growing populations. Reviewers writing in a preface to the 2013 edition of *Paleopathology and the Origins of Agriculture* (first written in 1984) noted:

> Human populations have pushed carrying capacity and required new technologies that were adopted as needed, not 'invented'. We know that many new technologies including those in food processing were understood long before they were implemented; the latter occurred only as need arose.[17]

Michael Pollan mentions three technologies, all associated with the preservation of foods: pickling, fermenting and smoking. Pickling can be dated back some 4,000 years where foods were allowed to ferment with what we now know as bacteria leading ultimately to the production of a food preserving acid (acetic acid) derived from the transformation of sugars into vinegar. In addition to its capacity as a method of preservation, pickling also introduced a highly sought after flavour and the bacteria, responsible for the sugar-to-acid transformation, also added to the nutritional value through its rich B vitamin concentration. The process of preserving foods by fermentation involves fruit and vegetable pickling but it also extends to other forms of food such as yogurt, which is preserved by the production of lactic acid from milk sugars or lactic acid from the sugars in finely chopped cabbage leading to sauerkraut. Salami and similar sausage like meats were preserved by mixing first with salt and then stored in airtight sections of animal gut for further transformation via fermentation. Finally, smoking probably started in caves where chunks of meat were hung to dry in air but were noticed to have a particularly attractive flavour where smoke permeated the atmosphere. Later, salting would be combined with smoking for a very efficient and tasty method of food preservation. Michael Pollan chooses these three forms of food preservation as evidence that man has always used processing in the food chain. It is what Michael Pollan leaves out that is most frustrating if not most disingenuous.

Let's take one of man's favourites: booze. It's been around for millennia. In an excellent paper on alcohol in Chinese culture, McGovern writing in the prestigious *Proceedings of the National Academy of Science* commented thus:

> Throughout history and around the world, human societies at every level of complexity discovered how to make fermented beverages from sugar sources available in their local habitats. This nearly universal phenomenon of fermented beverage production is explained by ethanol's combined analgesic, disinfectant, and profound mind-altering effects. Moreover, fermentation helps to preserve and enhance the nutritional value of foods and beverages. Because of their perceived pharmacological, nutritional, and sensory benefits, fermented beverages thus have played key roles in the development of human culture and techno-logy, contributing to the advance and intensification of agriculture, horticulture, and food-processing techniques. Among all strata of society, they have marked major life events, from birth to death, as well as victories, auspicious events, and harvests, etc. Rulers and 'upper class' individuals with leisure and resources particularly were drawn to feasting on a grand scale, which often featured special fermented beverages served in and drunk from special vessels. In their most developed form, such celebrations were formalized into secular or religious ceremonies for the society at large.[18]

So, we could eat grapes and enjoy their gastronomic properties and their nutritional value. Or, we could ferment them, forget about nutrition and enjoy the ensuing intoxicating and mind-altering properties of delectable wines.

If humans took to booze like ducks to water, they similarly took to sugar. An ancient rock painting in the Cave of the Spider near the Spanish port of Valencia dating back 12,000 years depicts a man collecting honey from a tree hive with bees buzzing all around him. Sugar as we know it today has its origins in India, in the fertile delta of the Ganges. According to the French food historian, Maguelonne Toussaint-Samat, the first mention of sugar in Indian literature is from the Sanskrit epic, *Ramayana*, which describes a banquet 'with tables laid with sweet things, syrup, canes, to chew . . .'[19] She goes on to point out that the first industrial plant for the manufacture of crystalline sugar from sugar cane was established by Arab merchants on the island of Crete, which in Arabic is known as *Qandi*, over more than a millennium ago. Thus sugar became known as Qandi sugar and that was eventually abbreviated in the US to the term 'candy'. The Arabs were to take the food processing of sugar cane further by converting the sugar to caramel, which is effectively what toffee is made of. Today caramel is the main component of the brown colour of all cola drinks. They also mastered the art of converting sugar cane pulp into a syrup and also treacle and the natives of north-east America tapped maple trees to yield a golden syrup. So, sugar and many versions of sugar processing are ancient, and in no way a modern invention.

There are many other examples of food processing, which emerged in the earliest stages of our agricultural existence, two of which I will briefly discuss. Grains are pretty nutritious but somewhat unappetising. The transformation of grains into bread was one of the most important innovations in the human food chain and bread became a symbol for many religions. Thus the ritual offering of food to the ancient Greek gods, *psadista* was made of bread, wine and oil. We know that flour was mixed with salt, water or milk and some oil to produce dough, which was cooked on hot stones to yield unleavened bread. How yeast came to play a role in bread making is unknown but like many culinary inventions, it's likely to have been an accidental occurrence, which was noticed and then copied by some observant and adventurous cook. Sweet cakes were also widely used incorporating sugar into the baking process and additional ingredients could include fruit, cream cheese or sesame seeds. Another major leap in food processing was the development of dairy produce such as butter, cheese and yogurt. In the modern food chain, milk is homogenised to blend the creamy top part with the rest of the milk. In times gone by, indeed in my childhood when homogenised milk was delivered in bottles to our doorstep, the cream, which floated to the top was decanted off for use in desserts with added sugar. In ancient times, the transport on horseback of such cream, stored in containers made from animal stomach, would have churned into butter leading ultimately to the development of mechanical churns, images of which date back to 2,000 BC. Unlike today's pasteurised milk, that of the ancients would have been in raw form and would have contained bacteria. Leaving milk in the heat would allow these bacteria to grow, thus creating acid conditions that would result in the formation of the solid curd and the liquid whey. Almost certainly the earliest dairying was with goats and sheep with dairy cows coming later. The solid curds could be salted, cooked, pressed to yield simple cheeses such as cream cheese or cottage cheese. In Mediterranean countries highly salted (brined) unfermented cheeses such as feta and halloumi were popular. Cheeses that were fermented and often left to mature for long periods were developed across Europe. The fermentation process required some form of yeast or mould and once again happenstance was the stimulus for particular local cheeses. Certain hard cheeses such as parmesan (officially called parmigiano-reggiano) were designed as a grated garnish to pasta or salad dishes. Processing of cheese even went as far as adding an artificial colour, even if the source of the colour was of natural origin. Red Leicester gets its red colour from the introduction of the colouring agent annatto, derived from the achiote tree. Finally, milk was processed to produce yogurt. The milk was subjected to mild heat to kill any existing bacteria and to ensure that the whey and casein (curd) proteins remained as a unit. Two types of bacteria were used to make the yogurt, one to ferment the milk sugar to lactic acid and another to impart the unique flavour of yoghurt. Many yoghurts, especially in Greece, were sweetened with honey.

One could go on and focus on the extraction of oils from seeds or the production of fast foods such as sausages and pizza. The former was dominated by local recipes with a generic composition of cheap pork cuts, pork offal, often blood with bread, salt and many different types of flavouring. Many had ancient regulations stretching back almost 800 years such as the Thuringian sausage, which still enjoys its unique marque under European law. Pizzas were available as cheap street food in Naples in the fifteenth century and were derived from garnished Greek pitta bread or focaccia. In the nineteenth century a special pizza was served to Queen Margherita of Italy with the colours of the Italian flag (red as in tomatoes, white as in mozzarella and green as in basil). Processed food is, quite simply, ancient and mostly designed not to enhance the nutritional quality of the food but to enhance its gastronomic and keeping qualities.

Milestone #5: Industrialisation

Processed food emerged fairly rapidly from the settled agricultural community and in the centuries that followed it was more a process of the refinement and development of these technologies. Some of the great innovations in man's food supply involved the mechanisation of farming, greatly increasing efficiency and reducing costs. Among the most important innovations that led to a huge boost in agricultural output was the discovery of the technology to allow ammonia-based nitrogenous fertilisers to be made synthetically, thus making the use of bird manure, such as from the Galapagos Islands, redundant. Two German chemists, Fritz Haber and Carl Bosch were to receive Nobel prizes for the discovery of these technologies.[20] Food preservation technologies were also major contributors to the increasing efficiency of the distribution of foods well beyond the point of production. In 1806, the Frenchman Nicolas Apert was awarded a prize from the French Navy for his invention of canning, a process that was first applied to the heat preservation of foods in glass bottles that were subsequently sealed. However, the fragile nature of glass soon led others to metal and another Frenchman, Philippe de Girard, working in Britain in 1810, invented the process of canning using tin. Again, the foods were heated under pressure and the tin can sealed with solder. The problem was, however, that opening these cans literally required a hammer and chisel so the technology only took off when a specialist in medical instruments by the name of Robert Yates invented the hand-held tin opener. These new technologies were not without their public suspicion. A main supplier to the navy by the name of Stephan Goldner was responsible for a shipment of tinned meat from Romania, which was found to be fraudulent requiring the destruction of 300 tons of the product. Goldner was also the purveyor of tinned food to the ill-fated Franklin Arctic expedition in which all were lost and, according to popular theory, it was the lead in the tinned food that was responsible. But, in the end, tinned food dominated and was constantly improved by the food giants of the time.

Refrigeration was also a major innovation that transformed the human food chain.[21] In the nineteenth century, ice was cut from frozen lakes using a horse-drawn ice plough and distributed to the great cities of America. In 1843, New Yorkers used 12,000 tons of ice. By 1856, this had shot up to over 100,000 tons. Whilst many industries had machines to make ice, these were very large, noisy and dangerous. It would take until the early part of the twentieth century for the domestic fridge to arrive with Kelvinator producing its Frigidaire domestic fridge in 1916. Clarence Birdseye developed the application of rapid freezing technologies, which would spawn the frozen food industry in 1924 and his company, the General Seafood Company, would eventually become Kraft General Foods.

Soft drinks were first dispensed in Paris as a non-carbonated drinks sweetened with sugar in the seventeenth century and, following the recognition by chemists that carbon dioxide was responsible for the bubbles in health spa waters, the first carbonated soft drinks emerged in the mid-eighteenth century. Soda fountains flourished in the US in the early part of the nineteenth century and in 1885, John Pemberton invented the first cola drink, which would eventually lead to the creation of the Coca-Cola Company. Just as the evolution of the tinned food industry awaited the advent of the tin opener, the soft drinks industry had to wait until someone invented a metal, sealable but easily removable bottle cap to sustain the pressure of the dissolved carbon dioxide.

Milestone #6: The High Street

If the industrial revolution was largely responsible for technologies that allowed food to be transported to areas far from their place of origin, the catering and retail sectors had to respond to the part of the supply and demand equation. Today when we walk into a Tesco store or a McDonald's fast food outlet, we expect to see a pretty standard layout wherever in the world we might be. There is a tendency to think that this is a recent concept and that in the past, all shops were unique to the proprietor. Whilst that is true to an extent, there was a very significant growth in the highly standardised retail and fast food stores. Fred Harvey was a British immigrant to the US who built up a chain of highly standardised restaurants and lunch counters along the Santa Fe railway and at his peak in the late nineteenth century, he had 65 such facilities as well as a dozen high-quality hotels.[22] The famous Harvey girls wore a standard uniform, served the meals and worked to the highest standard. Their lifestyle was captured forever in the 1946 MGM movie starring Judy Garland. Absolutely everything was standardised from the measure of tablecloths to the menu cycle, but all his hospitality was of the highest quality and keenest price. The retail outlets began to blossom. Home and Colonial stores began trading in 1883 and by 1900 had 100 premises expanding rapidly to 3,000 by 1903. Tesco started off with one store in 1924 and had expanded to 100 by 1939. Tesco, for those who like useless information derived its name from its first tea supplier: T. E. Scowell! Skaggs supermarkets claimed over 400 outlets in 1926 when it merged with Safeway to grow the combined number of outlets to almost 750 in one swoop. All of these stores exerted great power in the purchasing of foods and they greatly contributed to a cheaper and more diverse local food chain. All had standard layouts and all had a standard but proprietary style of retailing. A final innovation that didn't quite last was the automat where cold and hot food was dispensed from a wall of little boxes each opening after the appropriate sum was entered to yield a sandwich type meal. The automat became the butt of many jokes in the depression and today the automat is defunct and is replaced by specialist vending machines found in almost all airports, bus and railway stations, hospitals etc.

If indeed we want to find the root cause of the modern obesogenic environment, then we must look at the mass production of food, made possible by advances in everything from fertilisers, to mechanisation, to low fuel prices and beyond the production side of the food chain to its distribution via high throughput supermarkets with remarkable purchasing power who could send prices downwards such that only a few global brands could survive. You can blame the advent of McDonald's or Kentucky Fried Chicken or Coca-Cola or Mars bars. The reality is that recent food invention had relatively nothing new to contribute to the obesogenic food chain. It was mass production, mass distribution, mass branding and mass advertising. Sixteenth-century Aztec girls wore popcorn necklaces long before America was discovered.

Let me now remind you of what Michael Pollan wrote:

> It's true that foods have long been processed in order to preserve them, as when we pickle or ferment or smoke, but industrial processing aims to do much more than extend shelf life. Today foods are processed in ways specifically designed to sell us more food by pushing our evolutionary buttons-our inborn preferences for sweetness and fat and salt. These qualities are difficult to find in nature but cheap and easy for the food scientist to deploy, with the result that processing induces us to consume much more of these ecological rarities than is good for us.

Now let's go through a list of foods which together account for 90% of the caloric intake of the average Irish consumer. If I take bread, milk, cheese, yoghurt, butter, margarine, oils, eggs, potatoes, vegetables, fruits, nuts and meat, I have accounted for 61% of all calories. Where in that list do I find the type of modern addictive-type processed food that Pollan writes about? If I add in alcoholic beverages the figure rises to 68%. I could now add in breakfast cereals, biscuits, cakes, buns and pastries and the figure rises to 79%. Breakfast cereals are a nineteenth-century invention and biscuits are as old as cereal processing. In Tuscany, *cantucci* refers to a cake made with flour, sugar, eggs and almonds, baked for 20 or so minutes and then re-baked to cook it twice. This gives rise to the term biscuit from the word *biscotti*, twice cooked. So cakes, biscuits and pastries are an ancient invention and not that of a modern food scientist. Sugar intake brings the value to 81% and so we are left with: meat pies, meat rolls, sugar, chocolate and non-chocolate confectionery, savoury snacks, soups and sauces, and carbonated soft drinks. If I give half of these to the modern food scientist, then he or she has just 10% of all caloric intake as an absolute maximum. Blaming the modern food technologist for the obesity epidemic through the development and marketing of sugary, fatty and salty foods, is utterly false, useless but popular and simple. But it won't help us plan realistic strategies to tackle the national and global challenges of obesity. But assigning blame is fashionable today in the pell-mell to explain obesity. And when we move from foods to calories that fashion also exists. It is to the fashion of particular calories that we now turn.

CHAPTER FIVE

The Fashion of Culpable Calories

Identifying foods likely to lead to a healthy weight is an ancient practice dating back to the great Greek philosophers with the Hippocratic Oath II stating: 'I will apply dietetic measures for the benefit of my patients according to my ability and judgment.' Plato in particular had strong views on which foods would lead to a healthy diet, which with exercise, ensure optimal health. Foods that he encouraged were dairy products, cereals, honey, legumes and fish and foods that should be restricted included meat, confectionery, olive oil and wine.[1] We would wait until the seventeenth century for the first step in understanding energy or calories as we would come to know it by when Johann Becher proposed that combustible materials were rich in phlogiston, which he hypothesised was released during combustion. Antoine Lavoisier, in the late eighteenth century refuted this theory by demonstrating the association of oxygen and hydrogen in the generation of heat during combustion. The final major step to understanding this heat of combustion came from Nicolas Clément in the nineteenth century when the term calorie was defined. In time, the nature of our calorie-producing nutrients became known and the US scientist Wilbur Atwater in the late nineteenth and early twentieth century assigned calorific values to the energy-yielding nutrients, carbohydrate, fat, protein and alcohol and these values prevail to this day. Within the popular media, in diet books and blogs and to a limited extent in the scientific literature, debates take place on which sources of calories are best for health, including weight management. Alongside that, there is also a media avalanche of the foods which 'cause' obesity, most of which have the same rigors of experimental science as Plato, namely none. In this chapter, I want to look at the idea that some calories are more likely to promote weight gain or weight loss than others. At present, the media abounds in headline articles explaining the demise of fat as the big nutritional villain in obesity and its replacement by sugar. According to these media reports, there has been a climb-down by official agencies on the disadvantages of dietary fat. Nothing could be further from the truth. The confusion arises from a number of heavily criticised epidemiological studies that examined all the available evidence in the scientific literature to conclude that saturated fats are in fact not associated with a statistically increased risk of heart disease. These conclusions are not based on human intervention experiments but on statistical inferences. The dairy and meat industries were delighted with this news. So too were those scientists and commentators who regarded sugar as the 'new tobacco'. The absolute irrefutable fact is that nobody ever said that saturated fats or foods rich in saturated fats caused heart disease. What was said was that by modifying the nature of dietary fat or composition – a reduction in saturated fats and partial replacement with unsaturated fats – average blood cholesterol levels would be lowered. That assertion was based on a very large body of evidence, not based on epidemiology, but on direct human dietary intervention studies. In fact, I cannot think of an area of diet and health that is underpinned by experimental evidence anywhere near to the extent that the saturated fats–blood cholesterol link is built. Lowering the average level of blood cholesterol in a population, together with improved management of high blood pressure, a reduction in smoking and an increase in physical activity, would lead to lower rates of heart disease. That was proven to be the case and to reverse that advice on saturated fats, would be quite unethical, leading to a significant rise in heart disease. In fact, very recent and well planned dietary intervention studies, in which saturated fats were replaced by unsaturated fats, have again shown that changing dietary fats toward the standard dietary advice would lower deaths from heart disease by about 15 to 30%.[2&3] In this regard, nothing has changed in the last half-decade or more.

So how come we all went mad on a low fat spree? When dietary guidelines were first issued, the advice was to lower saturated fats (from about 20% of daily calories to 10%) and to partially replace them with unsaturated fats (from about 6 to 10% of daily calories). Total fat intake was recommended to fall from about 40% of calories to 35%. All of the reduction proposed in fat intake was focused on saturates. The modest reduction overall fat intake had the added benefit that it would make our diets less energy dense and thus help combat the emerging public health problem of obesity. So it wasn't mainstream science that set this low fat spree in motion. It was the media with the help of some scientists who advocated an extremely low fat intake. And they had an ally – the food industry. 'Low in fat' or 'Fat free' became their marketing catch cries and innovation after innovation brought total fat levels down. The same dietary advice that prevailed decades ago still prevails, more or less unchanged. However, the media, tired of the old story on fats found a new villain, sugar. It is a villain that has been around for a long time and it is to sugar we first turn to in considering the topic of fashionable calories.

As far back as 1670, it was recognised that the human frame was getting bigger and this led the French historian Jean-Louis Flandrin to refer to the development of a 'plumped up silhouette between the year 1450 and 1650' and in his view, this growth in body size was very definitely attributed to sugar.[4] Cakes, biscuits, sugary compotes and sweet liqueurs were all the rage and the famous seventeenth century pharmacist Moyse Charas noted that so great was the diversity and availability of such sugar-rich delicacies that 'if one wanted to stock all such preparations, the stores wouldn't be big enough to display them all.' Jean Anthelme Brillat-Savarin was an eighteenth-century French politician and lawyer but he was also arguably the father of modern gastronomy and epicureanism. His greatest work *Physiologie du Goût* (*The Physiology of Taste*) was published just months before his death. He famously stated: 'Tell me what you eat and I will tell you what you are.' He believed that all of the diet-related maladies of the time could be blamed on sugar and starch and he was a big proponent of protein. Of course, he did not have one scintilla of experimental evidence to back up this belief which makes him not so different from many of today's high priests of public health nutrition. Just about every generation has seen a popular proponent for the restriction of sugar intake: Sir Robert McCarrison (1878–1960) with his book *Studies in Deficiency Disease*,[5] Professor John Yudkin (1910–95) with his book *Pure White and Deadly*[6] and today's anti-sugar champion Professor Robert Lustig with his book *Fat Chance*.[7] Against that historical perspective, let's turn to the science of sugar and obesity.

Sugar, as most people know it, is derived from either of two sugar producing crops: sugar cane or sugar beet. The product is pulped, washed, the sugar extracted and then crystallised. It is sold to consumers for use in the household but the majority is sold into the food and catering industry. Sugar beet is primarily a European crop while sugar cane was a major crop of the West Indies, the Caribbean and particularly Cuba. The price of sugar cane is wide open to fluctuations due to climatic effects on yield and on variability in global demand. This economic or price uncertainty prompted the creation of a new source of sweetness in the diet, with the misnomer of high fructose corn syrup (HFCS). Thus, in 1974 and 1979–80, US and global sugar prices soared five-fold in two separate market peaks.[8] The advent of a new technology that could replace sugar with an identical alternative at a stable low price became a simple no-brainer. Sugar was priced out of the US markets with strict import quotas introduced in the early 1980s to maintain very high domestic sugar prices, double the global price. HFCS was to almost completely replace sugar in the US diet. The manufacture of HFCS is technically simple. Starch, which is a long multi-stranded chain of glucose units, is extracted from corn and industrial enzymes are then used to first break down the starch to glucose. Other industrial enzymes convert some of the glucose to fructose. The glucose and fructose can now be blended together and the most popular blend with consumers was 55% fructose and 45% glucose, an identical blend to that found in honey. For the US corn farmer and for the US government a switch to HFCS made huge sense.

So what happens when we drink a can of sugar-sweetened beverage? In the US, the 'sugar' will be HFCS.[9] In Europe it will be table sugar or sucrose as derived from sugar beet. Europe didn't embrace HFCS but supported in its social policy the local beet farmer. By EU law, the maximum of EU sugar supply as HFCS was limited to just 5%. Sucrose will be instantly digested to its two-component parts glucose and fructose, which are exactly what HFCS yields. Thus as far as our gut is concerned there is no difference between sucrose (50% glucose bound to 50% fructose) and HFCS (a blend of 45% glucose and 55% fructose. Glucose levels in the blood will rise immediately and will reach a peak about 30 minutes after starting to drink the sugar-sweetened beverage and by 60 minutes it will have returned to normal. As the level of glucose rises in the blood, insulin is released from the pancreas to distribute the glucose into fat and muscle. As the glucose levels fall back to normal, so too does the insulin. This post-prandial rise and fall of blood glucose applies to 85% of absorbed glucose. The remaining 15% goes to the liver for storage as a polymer of glucose known as glycogen. The fate of fructose is quite different. The fructose goes to the liver where about half is converted to glucose and released into blood. About a quarter enters the blood as lactic acid, which tissues such as muscles can use for energy. A fifth remains in the liver converted to glucose and retained in the liver as glycogen. Only 5% of the absorbed is converted to fat to be either stored in the liver or exported into blood. Herein lies the controversial interpretation of the data, which fuels the mass media and popular books in their view that sugar is toxic.

Whatever data might exist on fructose intake is of utterly no relevance to our understanding of diet and weight control since humans only consume fructose with glucose. So if the debate is between sugar (sucrose) and HFCS, let us turn to the opinions, not of individuals, but of expert committees who have considered this issue. The Council on Science and Public Health of the American Medical Association concluded:

Because the composition of HFCS and sucrose is so similar, particularly on absorption by the body, it appears unlikely that HFCS contributes more to obesity or other conditions than sucrose . . . At the present time, there is insufficient evidence to restrict the use of HFCS or other fructose-containing sweeteners in the food supply or to require the use of warning labels on products containing HFCS.[10]

The US Dietetics organisation's position paper on HFCS states:

By increasing palatability of nutrient-dense foods/beverages, sweeteners can promote diet healthfulness. Scientific evidence supports neither that intakes of nutritive sweeteners by themselves increase the risk of obesity nor that nutritive or nonnutritive sweeteners cause behavioral disorders.[11]

Turning away from the details of sugar and HFCS metabolism, what is the epidemiological evidence that nutritive sweeteners cause obesity? If there were a causal relationship, one would expect that the overall intake of nutritive sweeteners (sugars and HFCS) would parallel the rise in obesity. Well that just has not happened.[12] Between 1970 and 2000, US obesity rates rose by 250%. In contrast, total nutritive sweetener intake rose by about 20%. If you focus solely on HFCS you can see a dramatic rise in use over this period almost in parallel with obesity rates. However, as HFCS intake soared (due to levies on sugar imports) the intake of sucrose plummeted. The net effect was moderate rise (20%) in overall nutritive sweetener intakes. In Europe where HFCS is limited to 5% of the nutritive sweetener market, overweight and obesity rates have soared with no evidence of any rise in overall nutritive sweetener intake. In the UK for example, per capita intake of refined sugars fell from 126 g/head/d in 1963 to 99 g/head/d in 2003, during which time the Brits got quite fat. Here in Ireland, our sugar intake as a percentage of energy hasn't changed in over 20 years and again, we grew our national girth in that period.[13] So, should we restrict our intake of sugar to reduce the risk of obesity? Yes, if our caloric intake exceeds our caloric input and if the intake of sucrose is distorting our overall caloric intake. But that simple statement will also be made for starch, protein, fat and alcohol. Before leaving sucrose, it is worth noting that glucose in the blood, which is derived mainly from all dietary carbohydrates, is the only fuel used by the brain and the brain is an expensive organ in terms of energy needs. By weight, the brain accounts for no more than 2% of total body weight and yet, it consumes 20% of caloric intake, exclusively as glucose every day. So if an individual has an energy requirement per day of 2,000 calories and carbohydrates accounts for 40% of this energy that translates into 200 grams of carbohydrates. If the brain uses 20% of energy from glucose then that amounts to 100 grams of glucose. Thus our brains consume half of our entire glucose intake whether it comes from sugar or starch. There are some interesting observations on how sugars influence concentration. The brain uses only glucose as an energy store and doesn't use fats or proteins (or alcohol for that matter). Now evidence is emerging that mental fatigue is a reality and that food can not only overcome it but also change decision-making. In a paper in the prestigious journal, *The Proceedings of the National Academy of Science*, the decisions of judges in an Israeli court of appeal were studied.[14] Basically, favourable decisions as to parole review were at about 65% through the morning but fell to near zero before breaks and lunch, returning immediately to 65% after a break or meal. Other data shows that those who were given chocolate cookies to eat prior to a test fared far better that those who were shown the chocolate biscuits but who were asked to resist them and were given radishes to nibble on instead. The latter gave up after an average of eight minutes while those allowed the chocolate cookies kept going. Keeping the brain going is important and snacking helps.

Sugar and Fats Calories: Recent Lab Studies

So epidemiology tells us that the evidence against sugar and pro fat is built on a weak foundation. As ever, the ultimate move is to the experimental biologists. I want first to look at two fairly recent human nutrition interventions, one involving human volunteers living inside a human calorimeter or metabolic chamber, the other involving an intervention study among free-living individuals. First let me explain what exactly live-in calorimeters or metabolic chambers are. They are like medium size hotel rooms where people live for several weeks. They have a bed, a desk, a treadmill and toilet facilities and all dietary intake and physical activity are totally supervised and provided by the research team. The rate and nature of gaseous material (air) entering the chamber is extensively monitored. Loss of incoming oxygen and gain of outgoing carbon dioxide, together with energy losses in stools, are monitored and using fancy mathematics, the researchers can quantify the balance of and oxidation of fat, carbohydrate and protein in the food supplied. In addition in-room devices can monitor changes in body weight and body composition. So let's begin with the newer of these two studies.[15]

As already indicated, in recent years, it has become quite fashionable to argue that the real culprit in obesity is carbohydrates and as such fats have gained considerably good marks in the hierarchy of villainous calories. Gary Taubes, a highly influential author on this topic wrote thus: 'Any diet that succeeds does so because the dieter restricts fattening carbohydrates. Those who lose fat on a diet do so because of what they are not eating – the fattening carbohydrates.'[16] The carbohydrates are fundamentally turned into fat. All very well in theory but now, the results of an impeccably designed human study will greatly challenge this recent view that fats are good and carbohydrates are bad. Studies such as this are often criticised by epidemiologists who are accustomed to working with large numbers in a minimally invasive environment. Smaller studies extract huge amounts of biologically relevant material through high-tech, expensive and invasive studies. But fear not. All human studies are approved by a local ethics committee and these always demand researchers show that their chosen statistical sample is large enough to find an effect if one truly exists. So such knee-jerk criticisms are based on ignorance.

The volunteers were extremely obese. The males had a BMI of 38 while that of females was 33. The study randomised the subjects into one of two arms for 11 days of dietary intervention and all of this period was conducted in a metabolic chamber allowing strict measures of all aspects of calorimetry, with strict clinical supervision. For the first five days in each study arm, the subjects ate what is referred to as a eucaloric diet. That is, they received the exact amount of calories that they needed simply to neither gain nor lose weight. The nutritional composition of each subject's eucaloric diets was identical with 50% energy from carbohydrate, 35% from fat and 15% from protein. Only the quantity of overall weight-maintaining calories varied. For the next six days, their caloric intake was reduced by 30% either through a very low fat diet or a very low carbohydrate diet. There were no other changes in the composition of the calorie-reduced diets. The only foods available to the subjects were those prepared by the research team and all eating occasions were supervised. On days two and five of the eucaloric diet and on days one, four and six of the energy restricted diets, the subjects spent 23 consecutive hours inside the metabolic chamber. When the six days of dieting ended, the subjects took a two to four week break before resuming the same protocol but switching from the low fat arm to the low carbohydrate arm and vice versa. The main effects were as follows, as outlined by the authors:

Body fat loss was calculated as the difference between daily fat intake and net fat oxidation measured while residing in a metabolic chamber. Whereas carbohydrate restriction led to sustained increases in fat oxidation and loss of 53 g/day of body fat, fat oxidation was unchanged by fat restriction, leading to 89 g/day of fat loss, and was significantly greater than carbohydrate restriction.

Basically speaking, the most effective way to lose weight was to shed fat and Mr Taubes was wrong. More importantly, these recent data agree with a large body of literature on similar work with whole body calorimeters, typified by works from the Medical Research Council's Dunn Nutrition Lab in Cambridge UK back in the 1980s.[17] The detractors of this – and there are many – argue that the numbers are too small or that the study didn't last long enough. However, they are usually epidemiologists for whom extremely costly and invasive human research techniques are not the norm. Simple epidemiological measurements such as dietary intake are inexpensive, invasive and flawed. With metabolic chambers, asking humans to live in them for eight days with all sorts of inroads into their privacy such as toiletry habits and other such daily habits, with uncomfortable devices to be worn to collect this and that bio-output and with a surrounding of fancy laboratory equipment churning out highly accurate data minute after minute isn't easy. So no, we don't use large numbers but we use the right numbers as statistically guided, otherwise the data paper wouldn't get past the editor. No, these results like all results are imperfect but they tell us a lot of true facts. Calories are calories no matter where they come from.

Let me turn now to another lab-based recent study involving free-living subjects. The study was led by Professor Julie Lovegrove at the Hugh Sinclair Unit at Reading University who enjoys a huge international reputation in human dietary intervention studies.[18] The objective of the study was to see what happened if secretly you took sugar calories out of certain foods and replaced them with artificial sweeteners and bulking agents such that the foods looked, smelled, felt and tasted the same but differed only in sugar calories. Of the 62 grams of added sugar in the UK diet 37 grams, about 60%, is amenable to change. The foods where sugar could be substituted with calorie free alternatives were: breakfast cereals, baked beans, puddings, chocolate, sweet confectionary, sweet spreads, savoury sauces, condiments, soft drinks, fruit juice, yoghurt, ice cream and other milks. Of the 37 g/d of exchangeable added sugars normally consumed in the UK diet, those from soft drinks and sugars accounted for about half (15 g/d or 40% of total). The food group 'sugar, confectionary and preserves' accounted for 37% of exchangeable sugars. The study had a crossover design so that in the first phase half was assigned to a normal diet and half to the same diet but with sugar reduced. At the end of eight weeks' study, the subjects took a break from the experiment but four weeks later they returned to switch arms of the study. To ensure that the 50 participants didn't deliberately change their weight, they were told that the study was to see how changes in diets influenced aspects of heart disease. They were thus unaware that the true objective of the study was to see if reducing total added sugars in the diet would reduce overall energy intake and thus cause weight loss. The net result was clear-cut. There were no changes in body weight when a large quantity of added sugars was secretly removed from the diet. The authors concluded:

> We observed that when sugar-reduced foods and beverages were consumed as part of an habitual diet no significant change in body weight was observed. This was due to energy compensation; fat and protein intakes were both higher on the sugar-reduced diet when compared to the regular diet.

To many, these results are not surprising. The human body defends its existing weight quite effectively for long periods before permanent damage is done and a new permanent weight is established. It is important to note that in this study, subjects did not know that the objective actually involved weight loss. In others, the subjects knew that they were in a study of added sugar calories and weight control. Thus in one study, caloric intake fell by 9% over 18 months when intake of sugar-sweetened beverages was reduced by 27% and of course weight also fell, about 500 grams for each serving of sugar-sweetened soda per day over the 18 months.[19] Yet another study gave adult subjects high sugar or sugar free snacks – 2 grams per kilogram body weight per day with the rest of the food chosen according to taste and appetite.[20] Caloric intake soared with the sugar supplements (+22%) as did sugar intake (+150 g/d). Naturally, weight soared in the sugar-supplemented group in response to a higher caloric intake. The key is this: will shedding soda lead to a reduction in caloric intake in which case weight will be lost, or will shedding soda be compensated by higher caloric intake through fat and sugars resulting in no statistically significant weight loss. The certainty, with which this is answered in the media, bears no bearing on the scientific complexity of the issue. It would be wrong to say that there is definitive proof from intervention studies showing categorically that reducing total sugar intake always and at all times leads to a compensatory increase, in particularly fat intake, resulting in a constant energy intake and no weight change. Equally it would be absolutely wrong to simply assume that if sugar calories are shed, energy intake will fall. We know far less than is popularly assumed about this critically important point. This was made clear by the American Medical Association:

> At this time, there are insufficient data to determine conclusively whether the use of non-nutritive sweeteners to displace caloric sweeteners in beverages and foods reduces added sugars or carbohydrate intakes, or benefits appetite, energy balance, body weight, or cardio-metabolic risk factors. Limiting added sugars is an important strategy for supporting optimal nutrition and healthy weights, as concluded in the 2009 American Heart Association scientific statement 'Dietary Sugars Intake and Cardiovascular Health'.[21]

Equally, many of us who have followed the vagaries of what is known as the sugar–fat seesaw will not be surprised by the results. In almost every study that has been looked at across the globe, dietary fat and sugar move in opposite directions when expressed as percentage energy.[22] Protein and starch remain fairly constant but a fat-loving savoury tooth will do battle with a sweet-loving sweet tooth. In this instance the data are heavily stacked in favour of an inverse relationship between sugar and fat intakes. This inverse relationship is even true among highly sugar conscious, insulin-dependent diabetics under strict clinical control.[23]

In summary, to gain weight, eat more calories than are needed. To lose weight, eat fewer calories than are needed. Don't worry whether it's fat or sugar or wine you shed, just shed calories. As Dolly Parton said to the BBC presenter Michael Parkinson: 'Honey, if you want to lose weight, get your head out of the slop bucket.' No truer words were ever spoken about weight regulation! The bottom line is this: If you want to lose fat from the body, first lose it from the plate, but make sure that the caloric deficit of fat leads to an overall deficit of calories from the diet.

UK Government Report on Carbohydrates and Health

The UK Scientific Committee Advisory on Nutrition completed a report on diet and health in 2015 with a specific emphasis on carbohydrates.[24] It would be remiss of this author not to refer to this document. As regards the relative benefit of variation in total fat and carbohydrate on BMI, the report concludes:

> The trials do provide evidence that an energy-restricted higher carbohydrate, lower fat diet, as compared with a lower carbohydrate, higher fat diet, may be beneficial as a dietary strategy for reducing body mass index, but there is high heterogeneity between trials and the evidence is limited due to a relatively small number of trials. The hypothesis that diets higher in total carbohydrate cause weight gain is not supported by the evidence from randomised controlled trials considered in this review.

When the experts examined the specific role of sugar-sweetened beverages and foods on obesity it concluded:

> Randomised controlled trials conducted in adults indicate that increasing or decreasing the percentage of total dietary energy as sugars when consuming an *ad libitum* diet, either through the substitution of other macronutrient components or by replacing sugars with non-caloric sweeteners, leads to corresponding relative increases or decreases in energy intake. Evidence from trials conducted in children and adolescents indicates that consumption of sugar-sweetened beverages, as compared with non-calorically sweetened beverages, results in greater weight gain and increases in body mass index, however the evidence is limited to a small number of studies. The findings of these trials suggest that there is inadequate energy compensation (degree of voluntary reduction in intake of other foods or drinks), for energy delivered as sugar.

All of the data on sugar-sweetened beverages and children were based on three randomised controlled trials, while for adults, the data from nine randomised controlled trials were used. All in all, the language of the report is conservative and cautionary. In the context of this book, it is important to remember that this group was asked to look at all carbohydrates and sugar as factors in obesity. It wasn't asked to review the overall drivers of obesity in the UK, to make detailed comparisons on all macronutrients (to include carbohydrate, fat, protein and alcohol) or on all food sources, and it wasn't asked to probe the physiological and psychological drivers of obesity in the UK. Another group, the UK Obesity Task Force was asked to do that and we will address their conclusions in the final chapter.

Starch

I entered the term 'starchy foods' into the Google search engine and I got 908,000 results to consult, should I want to. When I entered the term 'sugary foods' I got 5,490,000 results. Clearly, for the general public, starch is not high on the list of concerns compared to sugar. Unlike sugar, starch is made solely of glucose with glucose molecules joined end to end in long filaments with a branching structure here and there. The main sources of starch in western diets are potatoes, bread, pasta and rice. Because of its molecular design, starch is often referred to as a complex carbohydrate and in general, healthy eating guidelines promote a high intake of complex carbohydrates. Dietary fibre, as we will shortly see, also falls into this category of complex carbohydrates. Fashionable diets such as the Atkins Diet, the Paleo Diet, the South Beach Diet, the Dukan Diet and so on, are all very popular that require a strict reduction in starchy food intake and collectively have led to an undeserved bad name for starchy foods. 'Cutting out carbs' is a very common knee-jerk approach to dieting. If one wanted to find a possible metabolic reason to paint a bad picture of dietary carbohydrates, it is that low fat, high carbohydrate diets cause alterations in blood lipid profiles leading to an accumulation of so-called bad lipids and a decrease in so-called good lipids. However, the generally accepted dietary advice calls for a modest reduction in fat intake with a modest rise in starch intake, which should be compensated for by a reduction in the intake of sugars. So, if dietary advice is adhered to, the overall effect will be a beneficial effect on blood lipids.

Starch has entered the issue of obesity through a different route – that of the glycaemic index and glycaemic loads of individual foods. The glycaemic index of a food is determined as follows. Using a minimum of ten volunteers, an amount of the test food is eaten which will provide 50 grams of absorbable carbohydrate. Blood glucose is monitored over a two-hour period. The same ten volunteers on a separate occasion also consume 50 grams of pure glucose and again the blood glucose levels are monitored over a two-hour period. The overall glucose response in the test food is then related to that of the pure glucose and a value for the glycaemic index is calculated. Foods that rapidly release glucose into the blood stream have a high value on a range of zero to 100. Foods with slow release carbohydrates have lower values. The glycaemic load of a food is the glycaemic index multiplied by the expected total carbohydrate in a typical serving of a food. Although fast release carbohydrates are considered inferior to diets with slow release carbohydrates, the evidence for a role in obesity is not very strong. All aspects of the glycaemic index, load and response was considered by the International Carbohydrate Quality Consortium.[25] It concluded:

> Given the high prevalence diabetes and pre-diabetes worldwide and the consistency of the scientific evidence reviewed the expert panel confirmed an urgent need to communicate information GI and GL to the general public and health professionals, through channels such as national dietary guidelines, food composition tables and food labels.

Starches are associated with complex carbohydrates and fibre is often included in that definition. We will return to dietary fibre in chapter nine.

Alcohol

When we were young and on the rare occasions that we would eat out at a restaurant, the waiter would ask my father if he would like 'table wine'. You see, as a young family in the Catholic tradition, the only other wine that we would know of would be 'altar wine'. Not so today where alcohol is ubiquitous in society. Each gram of alcohol contains six calories while that of carbohydrate is four and that of fat is nine. So if alcohol is more available in modern society, then surely it must contribute to obesity. However, if respondents are inclined to under-report energy intake, they are for sure likely to under-report alcohol intake, certainly at the upper levels. The net effect is that there is literally little known of the links between alcohol intake and obesity. We know that liver disease is one of the most rapidly rising diseases of modern developed societies, which strongly suggests that it should be linked to a rise in obesity. However, the data are very limited and quite confusing when it comes to alcohol and obesity.

In this chapter we have looked at culpable calories, in particular sugars and fat. The bottom line is simple: all calories are equal and all will help you gain or lose weight at comparable rates. The time has now come to look at what we normally eat in terms of food choice to which the next chapter is devoted, beginning with the genetic regulation of our food choice.

CHAPTER SIX

Obesity: The Nature versus Nurture Debate

The predisposition to corpulency varies in different persons. In some it exists to such an extent, that a considerable secretion of fat will take place not with-standing strict attention to the habits of life and undeviating moderation in the gratification of appetite. Such predisposition is often hereditary.

(William Wadd, 1816)[1]

The next thing to be done was to consider why some are more susceptible to fat and liable to corpulency than others. The reasons whereof I presume to be . . . Others on the contrary have such flexible, lax and dilatable fibers that even temperance, exercise, study, abstinence and abridgment of rest and sleep cannot prevent corpulency although they eat and drink no more than what is required to answer the necessary demands of life.

(Thomas Short, 1828)[2]

In September 2006, I was honoured to give the opening plenary lecture to the first World Congress of Public Health Nutrition in the wonderful city of Barcelona. I was asked to talk on my choice of hot topics in the field and I chose four: vitamin D and the metabolic syndrome, the gut microflora and health, energy under-reporting in dietary surveys and the genetics of obesity, the subject of this chapter. When the question and answer session opened, there was a rush to the microphone from the great and good of public health nutrition, united in denouncing my case for a role, a significant role, of genetics in obesity. Their logic was thus: whether the present obesity epidemic started 50 years ago or 150 years ago, it remains a simple fact that in that period our genes have not changed one iota. The environment has changed and thus it is absurd to suggest that genes play a role in the present epidemic of obesity. It's the environment that has changed dramatically, leading to an abundant supply of cheap foods high in sugar, fat and salt, and that alone is the cause of obesity. In the course of this chapter, I will show that this is palpably wrong. However, I understand the sensitivity of public health nutrition to the intrusion of genetics into this arena. From their point of view, to admit that genes play a significant role in obesity, is to invite the overweight and obese population to throw their arms in the air and declare: 'It's not my fault. It's my genes.' Thus the strength of the argument that excess body weight is based on bad lifestyle choices would be diluted. It is an understandable position if it were true that genes play little or no role in obesity. However if genes do play a significant role in overweight and obesity, it is the duty of science to pursue that truth and hopefully exploit the attendant knowledge to help prevent obesity. Thus if we could arrive at a point in time where a genetic test could not only predict a predisposition to obesity but also to map out the main lifestyle choices to be avoided to prevent obesity, then we could tailor public health nutrition advice to a personalised genetic agenda. That day will come and although we are by no means near that day at present, we can see the road map that will bring us there.

Within a week of birth, all newborn babies are subject to a blood test derived from a heel prick, which is used to scan for high levels of certain compounds in blood. If a high level of a given metabolite is detected, alarm bells ring to indicate that the child might have a genetic disorder that could seriously compromise health. This test, known as the Guthrie test after its founder the US physician Robert Guthrie, screens for a number of genetically based disorders such as phenylketonuria (PKU), sickle cell disease and cystic fibrosis.[3] In the case of PKU, the test might reveal a high level of the amino acid phenylalanine in blood, indicative of a fault at the level of a single gene that carries the genetic code for this enzyme, which breaks down the amino acid, phenylalanine. If untreated, it can lead to mental retardation. However, a lifetime diet to manage blood levels of phenylalanine will completely normalise mental and cognitive function. This is an example of a genetic test that can indicate an impending problem and can then map out a lifetime solution to the problem. PKU is a monogenetic disorder in that one very specific gene totally fails to function. This will never apply to obesity, which has so many possible causes and complications that it is in contrast a polygenetic disorder, involving a small input from a multitude of gene. How therefore do we go about exploring the role of genetics in obesity? In the modern world of high-tech molecular biology, the gene-jockeys burrow downwards into the human genome to seek explanations. However, the most compelling evidence for a role of genetics in obesity dates back some 40 years to the study of identical and non-identical twins. However, before visiting the evidence from twins, it is wise to consider the very small number of very rare conditions where a single gene causes obesity.

Known Gene Defects and Clinical Conditions Involving Obesity

Many years ago, experiments were conducted with mice where parts of their brain involved with food intake were inactivated with the result that they overate and became obese. When these obese mice were surgically conjoined via their blood circulation with normal healthy mice, their obesity disappeared. This suggested that something was carried in blood, which interacted with appetite control signals to restore appetite to normal. To date, many such candidate regulatory signals have been identified, the first of which was the protein leptin, so named after the Greek word for thin, *leptos*.[4] Researchers at Addenbrooke's Hospital in Cambridge, UK have pioneered the use of leptin injections to cure a form of obesity in which the gene encoding the structure of leptin, or the gene for the synthesis of the receptor that binds leptin, are completely malfunctioning.[5] The consequence of the absence of leptin is the rapid development of severe childhood obesity due to over-consumption of food. So strong is the drive for food that children can become extremely aggressive when denied food. Thus a simple blood test that shows an undetectable level of leptin can lead to the successful treatment of this very rare condition, which affects about 1% of very severely obese subjects. Another example of a single gene defect is what is known as the Prader-Willi Syndrome (PWS) where a region of chromosome 15 is deleted. PWS has a frequency of 1 in 25,000 and is characterised by a voracious appetite leading to obesity.[6] Some researchers believe that the gut-produced and eating stimulating hormone, ghrelin, might be involved since levels of this hormone are elevated five-fold in PWS sufferers. However, whether this is a direct cause or a side effect of another cause remains unknown. There are many other examples of single gene defects or defects involving several genes that explain some very rare conditions of obesity. However, for the vast majority of obese and overweight humans, the genetic basis involves the combined impact of a small effect from a multitude of genes. The strength of that evidence comes from twin studies.

Twin Studies and the Genetics of Obesity

Twin studies play a major role in the determination of those characteristics that are highly heritable from the DNA that our parents give us. The genes we inherit from our parents constitute our genotype. Ultimately, those genes materialise in eye colour, height, blood cholesterol, personality, IQ, and all other measurable characteristics of a given individual and these collectively are referred to as our phenotype (after the Greek word '*phainein*', meaning 'to show'). Genes shape certain aspects of our phenotype such as the colour of our eyes while our genes and our environment jointly set others. Thus some people are born with naturally high levels of blood cholesterol while others attain a high level of blood cholesterol partly through genetic factors but to a considerable extent due to the nutritional aspect of their environment. The relative importance of the role of genes and the role of the environment can easily be distinguished within twin studies. All twins share the same environment before birth and most share the same environment for long periods after they are born, right up to adulthood when they leave home and go their separate ways. However, identical twins share one key element that non-identical twins don't share, namely their genome. Identical twins have identical genomes while non-identical twins have a genome that is as variable as that between non-twin brothers and sisters.

Twin studies on obesity were first carried out in the 1980s and since then over 500 such studies have been reported in the scientific literature. The early studies showed that approximately 70–80% of the variability in obesity could be explained by genetic factors. Before pursuing this further with more modern evidence, let me explain what this means. If you travel around your local town or city, you will see some people who are very severely obese, almost finding it quite difficult to walk. You will see others that are not quite obese, others that are quite overweight and others that are simply a little plump. But you will also see people who are not at all overweight and you will even see some skinny folk. Now all these people live in the same environment and are equally exposed to the obesogenic aspects of that environment. And, within that same environment, we have a spectrum of body weights from slim to obese. It is primarily our genes that determine which part of this spectrum we will fall on. But, if you could remove the obesogenic environment, if you could curtail the wide availability of cheap palatable foods laced with the usual suspects of fat, sugar and salt, then obesity would vanish and genes just wouldn't count any more. But in the highly obesogenic environment we live in, it is our genes which determine where we are placed in the obesity league table.

Whenever I talk about genes and obesity to a lay audience, the resistance to the genetic truth emanates from two very commonly held prejudices. The first is that obesity is mainly a problem of the less economically well off or those with little education. So when you look around your town or city, the obese overweight persons are far more likely to be less well off and poorly educated. Take a stroll through a shopping mall in a poor neighbourhood and you will see the spectrum of obesity from lean to obese. Take a similar walk in a mall in a well off district and you will see the same spectrum. It may well be that in the less well off mall there are more seriously overweight and fewer very lean. This we will explore in detail later in chapter 9. So the gene-led spectrum of weight distribution is seen in all socio-economic groups. The second prejudice is that of behaviour. Again, we will look at this in greater detail later but in this discussion on nature and nurture, we need also to scotch this prejudice. Take just one of these behavioural prejudices, that the obese have a low level of self-control. Thus the argument is that when I look around me, those overweight and obese people I see are actually just unable to control themselves. So what if that was true? Is it possible that poor self-control has both a genetic and an environmental dimension such as poor self-control learned from parental or familial behaviour? So the spectrum of genetically determined body weight is not marked by mere poor self-control. Are all gamblers fat? Are all alcoholics or smokers fat? Not at all.

Returning now to the inescapable evidence that obesity is a highly heritable trait, we move in time from the 1980s to the present. Bearing in mind that the 1980s is argued by some, wrongly as it is, as the starting point of the modern epidemic of obesity, maybe these early twin studies missed out on the huge growth in the obesogenic nature of our environment which we have seen in recent times. Endless numbers of recent studies have upheld the earlier twin studies that obesity had a heritability of somewhere around 70–80%. I would like to highlight two such studies. The first comes from the late Professor Jane Wardle of University College London.[7] She examined BMI and waist circumference in a sample of 5,092 twin pairs aged eight to eleven years of which 36% were identical twin pairs with 64% as non-identical twin pairs. Genetic factors explained 77% of the variation in BMI and 76% in waist circumference. For BMI, the environment accounted for 23% of the variation of which the 'shared' environment accounted for 10% of variability and 13% of the non-shared variability. Basically speaking, the shared environment refers to the home while the non-shared environment refers to different schools, sports interests, hobbies and the like. The shared and non-shared environment variability for waist circumference was broadly similar.

The second study I want to refer to is from an international collaborative project that pooled data on the heritability of obesity allowing a powerful analysis of the role of genetics from birth to adulthood.[8] Data from 23 twin birth cohorts in Canada, Sweden, Denmark and Australia were used with 12,018 twin pairs included. In all of these cohorts, twins were followed from birth to 19 years of age. At birth, the heritability of BMI was very low at about 7%. However, by five months of age, BMI had reached a heritability of about 50% and by year one, that figure had reached 80–90%. It hovered within that range of heritability right through to age 19 years with a dip to about 60% at age four and age seven years. These are extremely robust data because the same children were followed for about 19 years and the sample size was very large. A weakness is that the weight and height data were self-reported by parents and not directly measured by objective researchers. Nonetheless, the study remains a very important one. Whereas this study pooled all the data from different studies, another important paper reviewed all of the literature on twin studies. A significant finding of this review was that the variation across studies was greatest with smaller numbers of twin sets. Thus where the number of identical twins was less than 100 twin pairs, the correlations between identical twins ranged from 0.5 to 0.9. In correlation statistics, a value of zero indicates absolutely no correlations while a value of 1.0 indicates a perfect correlation. However, when the numbers of twin pairs in the studies under consideration reached 200, the correlation was in or around 0.8 across all studies. Another important set of statistics to emerge from this review was the correlation data for different groups. For identical twins, BMI showed a correlation of 0.74 between one identical twin and their sibling. For non-identical twins, this fell to 0.32 and for siblings, it fell further to 0.29. The parent–child correlation was 0.19 and the inter-spouse correlation was 0.12. Thus as the similarity of genetic makeup diminished so too did the correlations within a group. All in all, twin data show that the heritability of obesity is about 70–80%.

In addition to these quite simple studies of body weight heritability in twins, there are two other approaches to understanding this phenomenon. One is to study the heritability of twins reared apart. If the environment is more powerful than the estimates using twins raised together, then we should see this in such studies where identical and non-identical twins share radically different environments. One such study used a Swedish twin registry established over the period

1886 to 1958.[9] Of the 25,000 twin pairs, a total of 93 identical twins and 218 non-identical twins were reared apart. Their average age was 59 years and this represented individuals born at the turn of the last century when economic times were hard. The reasons for sending the twins for adoption were partly due to these economic difficulties and partly due to parental death or serious illness and the average age of separation of twins from their parents was 2.8 years. To complete the study, age- and BMI-matched twins that were reared together were also included. The inter-pair correlation of BMI for identical twins reared apart was 0.68. For those reared together, the value was almost identical at 0.70. For the non-identical twins, the values were lower at 0.20 for such twins reared apart and slightly higher at 0.30 for non-identical twins raised together. It should be noted that the age gap between separation was all of 56 years so the twins raised apart had a lifetime of different environmental influences and still, with the identical twins, their genes dominated their body weight in their sixth decade of life. This is just one of several studies of the heritability of BMI in twins raised apart and they all show a broadly similar finding. In a final area of this approach, the heritability of body weight relates to the extent to which adopted children compare with their biological and their adoptive parents.[10] All such studies have shown that children's weight correlates better with their biological parents than with their adoptive parents and this has also been found in studies of adoptees in adulthood.

One of the criticisms that could be laid at all of the above twin studies is that they show very strong associations between a person's genetic makeup and their body weight but that such associations don't really prove anything. To achieve that, one has to carry out some sort of experiment to test a given hypothesis. In 1990, the results of a long-term overfeeding study in identical twins were published.[11] Twelve pairs of identical twins with an average age of 21 were overfed by 1,000 kilocalories per day for six days a week for 100 days. The men were housed in a private dormitory and were under 24-hour supervision. The average weight gain was 8.1 kilograms but the range of weight gain was from 4.3 to 13.3 kilograms. The hypothesis that was to be tested in this study was effectively that although the 12 pairs of twins would show very different levels of response to the overfeeding, each identical twin would react very similarly to its twin. And that is what happened. The variation across the 12 pairs of twins was seven times greater than the variation between each twin pair. Thus some identical twins gained relatively little weight in this hyper-obesogenic environment while others showed a very high sensitivity to weight gain bringing us back to the common spectrum of weight distribution in the general population within a common environment. A second study was completed in which pairs of identical twins were put into a negative energy balance with weight loss induced by twice-daily bouts of exercise on a cycle ergometer.[12] Once again, identical twins behaved the same in respect of weight loss while across twin pairs, weight loss ranged from a loss of just over 8 kilograms to a loss of just 1 kilogram.

It is clear from these twin studies that in an obesogenic environment, which characterises the lifestyle of most modern economies, our individual position on the obesity league table is very much determined by genes. Take away the obesogenic environment, then you take away obesity and the role of genes therein. However, whilst we might tinker with this obesogenic environment, it is unlikely to vanish overnight. In the meantime, science will pursue a greater understanding of the role of genetics in obesity such that we will be better able to help individuals shape their own environment to minimise the risk of serious weight gain. Obesity arises from a plethora of areas from food choice to resilience, from the metabolism of adipose tissue to the nervous system. In the 1980s and 1990s when twin studies took off, the heritability of obesity was accompanied by studies of the heritability of certain elements of energy metabolism such as resting metabolic rate, waist circumference, subcutaneous fat as measured by skinfold thickness, the thermic effect of food, caloric intake, physical activity and so on. In some cases the heritability was significant such as in subcutaneous fat (44%) and resting metabolic rate (40–80%), but many of these measures have a high error level in measurement and thus it is difficult to sort out the wheat from the chaff. For example, estimates of habitual nutrient intake show very large day-to-day fluctuations and thus a single measure of nutrient intake is fraught with error. Even if we could measure with accuracy many of these elements of energy metabolism, each is itself composed of very many elements and sub-elements that unravelling the responsible genetic area is a huge challenge. For example, resting metabolic rate, which accounts for 70% or more of all energy expended daily, is determined by the total amount of fat in the body, the ratio of fat to lean mass and certain circulating hormones such as the thyroid hormone thyroxine. In turn, the levels of the thyroid hormone in blood are themselves determined by many factors so the pyramid of candidate causal factors grows ever larger. The search for a greater understanding of the nature of the heritability of obesity is now focused on specific genes on specific chromosomes.

Genes and Obesity

Proteins are the key regulatory mechanisms in the body. The protein insulin regulates blood glucose. The protein haemoglobin determines how much oxygen the blood can carry and the protein, thyroxine, plays a key regulatory role in energy metabolism. Each of these proteins is comprised of a chain of amino acids and the sequence of the amino acids determines the function of the protein. If there is a change to that sequence of amino acids, the function may now vary either to a more efficient or a less efficient plane. A segment or joint segments of our genetic code in DNA determine each protein. Again, DNA is a chain of just four repeating units called nucleotides: cytosine, guanine, adenine and thymine. The building blocks of the proteins, the amino acids, each have a defined sequence of any three of these nucleotide. Each combination of three nucleotides codes for just one amino acid.

Variation involving one nucleotide in each bundle of three is known as a single nucleotide polymorphism (SNP) pronounced 'snip'. You can inherit the normal variety of the DNA sequence from both parents or you might inherit one form of the SNP from one parent and the other form of SNP from the other parent. With today's technology, your entire genome can be searched for SNPs which vary from the dominant type. Thus the approach adopted by the gene-jockeys is thus. We can *a priori* identify a gene that we suspect (hypothesise) is higher in one condition, e.g. obesity, as opposed to another, e.g. normal weight, or we can search the entire genome for all 'snips' which are higher among the obese than in the lean. A number of genes have been identified using these techniques. The so-called FTO[13] gene has two versions and if you happen to inherit the two 'bad' versions from both parents, you will be about 4 kilograms heavier, on average, than say your sister who was lucky enough to inherit both the good versions. At present, there is great interest in the FTO gene. The second approach now seeks to identify all the SNPs that differentiate the lean and obese. Thousands of SNPs will be encountered but to reduce it to manageable levels, researchers take maybe the 30–50 that have the highest penetrance within the obese genome. The study populations are huge (>300,000) and of the near 100 or so important SNPs observed between the lean and obese, a total of 2.7% of variation in BMI can be explained. The more of the obesity risk SNPs an individual has, the greater their BMI. The problem is that when you hit the group, which has inherited the highest number of high-risk SNPs, we are talking about a sample of just ten out of the original 300,000 or so, a hit of just one in 35,000.

All of these data tell us that there is a needle in the haystack and we will need to learn a lot about the architecture of the haystack and the properties of the needle before any great breakthrough is made. But be warned. The press machines of universities will, from time to time, pepper the headlines which 'breakthroughs'. Read with a sceptical mind. As it stands, there are interesting genes to 'play around with' and we maybe learn something from their study. But the reality is that modern obesity is determined by a multitude of genes each making a small contribution. It is no longer enough to carry out gene studies on something as biologically crude as obese versus lean. Can we begin to look at the differential genetics of those who are obese with a higher as opposed to a lower sensitivity to the external cues of the modern food chain or those with fast versus slow eating habits? These may be more difficult to do but sending rockets into space isn't cheap.

We will return to genetics and obesity but in the specific context of food choice, a most fascinating area to which we now turn.

CHAPTER SEVEN

Regulating Food Intake: The Eyes Have It

In the movie, *Cool Hand Luke*, the prisoner hero, Luke, played by Paul Newman, makes a wager with his warders that he can eat 50 hard-boiled eggs in one hour. He succeeds but only with considerable help from his cellmates. Competitive or speed eating events are popular in the US where anything from hot dogs to ham and eggs are the foods to gorge upon. Leaving aside the frivolity of overeating contests, almost nobody wakes up one morning resolving henceforth to overeat and become fat. When people gain weight and become fat, it is generally involuntary. Somehow, over time, their energy intake has exceeded their body's needs for calories resulting in the slow and imperceptible addition of ounce after ounce, gram after gram of body fat until one day, the belt is too tight, the dress is no longer loose and hey presto, you're fat. How is it possible for some to fail to regulate appetite properly, that is, to eat to maintain a stable body weight, neither gaining nor losing body fat? That is the single most important question about obesity.

In this context, it is important to note that the term appetite refers both to the desire to eat and also the decision to stop eating. In other words, appetite represents the full spectrum from hunger to satiety. So complex is the subject of appetite that no one explanation will ever prevail. Rather there will be multiple routes to control appetite and thus multiple explanations as to why people passively overeat and gain weight. There are three broad areas in the regulation of food intake we need to consider. The first is the attributes of a food or meal that influences our appetite. The second addresses the biology of appetite. Finally, we need to consider the psychological and behavioural aspects of eating.

The first thing one needs to consider in the area of food choice and food intake is our varying tastes and preferences. I am unlikely to choose a food I don't like or to eat heartily on some dish I'm not so mad about. In fact, these days, guests are often asked about food preferences when invited to dinner. One might not like seafood. Another might dislike hot curries and another might not be overly fond of mushrooms. To begin to understand what makes foods attractive to some but not others, we need to consider the five senses of sight, taste, smell, touch, and hearing and how they relate to our experience with foods.[1]

Sensory Aspects of Food

Food has an appearance which involves the first sense, that of sight. Chefs go to great lengths to construct meals into visual masterpieces and the simple garnishing of a poached egg on toast with parsley will considerably improve its appeal. A dish that doesn't reach a certain acceptable level of appearance will fall down in its appetising appeal. I experienced the power of appearance in determining the acceptability of a meal when I dined in the Unsicht Bar in Berlin, best translated into English as the 'Blind Bar'. Your blind waiter who will sit you at your table collects you from a well-lit reception area where you choose menus and order drinks and then he or she leads you as a human train with hands on shoulders, through a chicane of black alleyways to a noisy and bustling restaurant. It is dark beyond belief where everything from floor to ceiling, from table to chair, from knife to fork and from cup to glass is black. With your eyes wide open, it's as dark an experience as you can ever have encountered. You are asked in advance to choose a broad menu: meat or fish or vegetarian or a surprise, but you do not know exactly what will be presented. We debated as to whether the starter was a cheese, possibly mozzarella, or chicken and whether the main course was pork or lamb. We got it wrong on both accounts. The visual dimension of food is incredibly powerful and it takes dinner at the Unsicht Bar to realise how powerful it really is.

After appearance comes flavour as the second sensory property and there are three elements to flavour. There is the taste which can be salty, sweet, bitter, sour or umami. Thus we can describe a soup as being very salty, a dessert wine as very sweet, a rhubarb pie as very bitter, a yoghurt as very sour and a Chinese dish with monosodium glutamate as having a meaty or umami taste. Flavour goes beyond taste because it also embraces odour. There is a definite smell in a bakery, a different one in a cheese manufacturing unit, a different one in a brewery or in a coffee house and individual dishes need a fine balance of all these odours to meet our expectations. Very often we ascribe the sensory properties of a food to taste when in fact it's the release of odours in the mouth, which waft up to the odour sensing cells in the nose that counts. Food loses its flavour when you have a cold and it's not because your taste buds are malfunctioning. It's your stuffed-up nose which is the problem because three quarters of what we think is taste actually comes from our sense of smell. So odour and taste are important but there is a third element to flavour and that is associated with the trigeminal nerve complex of the nose and mouth. Hot spicy foods stimulate our senses by causing very mild pain, irritating the soft linings of the nose and palate, which is transmitted to the brain by the trigeminal nerve complex. In contrast to foods that are hot and spicy, foods containing menthol sooth our palates and noses and fizzy drinks like champagne physically irritate these regions. So the trigeminal effect is a physical aspect of flavour transmitted to the brain. Finally, there is texture. You expect a fresh stick of celery to crunch in your mouth giving it a biting sensation you would not get with soup and you also expect to hear the crunch of the celery stick when you bite into it. Thus it embraces the senses of touch and hearing.

All of these attributes of foods are taken into account in the learning process that results in our list of foods we love, we hate and we are largely indifferent to. But that liking for a food is not finite. When Luke of *Cool Hand Luke*, ate his first boiled egg, it might have tasted quite nice. But by the third or fourth egg, that attraction of taste, flavour and the like that accompanied the first promptly disappears. This is a very well established phenomenon known as 'sensory specific satiety' which basically states that the more of a given food one consumes, the greater the decline in its sensory attraction.[2] Indeed, research shows that one doesn't even have to eat the food to see its attraction diminish. Just thinking about it can also work to induce sensory specific satiety. In one study, subjects imagined eating cheese cubes three times or 30 times and were subsequently given access to as many cheese cubes as they would like to eat.[3] Those who imagined eating cheese cubes 30 times subsequently consumed only half the amount of cheese compared to those who imagined cheese consumption only three times. The more often the consumption of the food was imagined, the less was subsequently eaten. When the same groups had free access to the confectionery brand M&Ms, no difference in M&M intake was seen. However when the intake of M&Ms was imagined 30 times, the subsequent intake of M&Ms fell to half that consumed by the group who imagined M&M intake only three times. So the more of a food we eat during a meal, the less attractive it becomes. Moreover, the more we dream about a food prior to a meal, the less of it we will eat. This phenomenon of sensory specific satiety might explain a common gastronomic practice across many cultures where a meal is made of many dishes. A starter of soup is fine because it is finite and not repeated as is the main course. Then, with a totally different flavour and taste comes dessert followed by cheese and coffee. Each course is enough to interest and satisfy the consumer's hedonic or pleasurable needs but not so big as to disrupt our appetite. Each new course sustains our hedonic interest. The serving of meals with multiple dishes is commonplace across the globe within different gastronomic traditions. In contrast, the fox eats what is there to satiety and doesn't seek different courses.

Taste is centrally important in food choice but it doesn't really help us to understand the sensation of hunger and of satiety and their derangement in passive overeating. Taste may tell us what we would like to eat. But something else drives the answer to the question: 'How much should I put on my plate to eat and/or how much might I leave on my plate when I'm full?' Thus we move from the qualitative side of food choice to the quantitative side.

In looking at this complex problem, there are two apparently opposite approaches that can be made to understand passive overeating. One is dominated by the biological sciences, the other by the behavioural sciences. Consider the following two quotes taken from important reviews on the subject. The first is from a group at the University of Cincinnati in the US: 'While we often think that when we put down our fork, it is a conscious decision. The reality is that ingestive behaviour is orchestrated by a wide range of biological signals that greatly impact on how much we eat.'[4] This group sees different foods and meals stimulating a set of biological processes governing hunger and satiety and thereby influencing how much we eat. Consider now a second quote from a group at the University of Bristol in the UK: 'Again, this distinction reinforces the notion that humans differ from other species because our meal size tends to be determined before meal onset rather than via feedback that is generated as a meal progresses.'[5] This view emphasises an *a priori* role for cognitive and behavioural processes rather than some biological pathway. In the course of this chapter, each of these competing elements will be explored, not with the intention of declaring the winner in the 'what controls hunger and satiety competition' but to provide an appreciation of the complexity of this central question as to the causes of obesity.

When I was a young undergraduate student, the regulation of food intake was a hot and fascinating topic and it still is today. Back then we knew that there was a specific region of the brain that was involved in regulating food intake. If the one side of this region (the hypothalamus) was deliberately damaged, rats became anorectic with no interest in food, eventually dying from self-imposed starvation. If the other half was deliberately damaged, the rats ate voraciously and rapidly became grossly obese. Clearly, there was something in the hypothalamus region of the brain which when stimulated by some biological signal switched on the desire to eat or switched on the sensation of satiety. The actual biological signals were unknown at the time but certainly both the hormone insulin and the blood metabolite it regulated, blood glucose, were held to play a central role. Today, these signals are much better understood and there is an array of hormones (leptin, ghrelin, peptide YY etc.) secreted mainly by the gut (the point of entry of food) and adipose tissue (the main reserve of energy in the body).[6] To focus on any one is like listening to the string or wind section of an orchestra playing its particular role in some great symphony. The reality is that these various hormones and signalling agents, known and yet to be known, act together to orchestrate the feeling of hunger and satiety. In this context, the term 'feeling' is very deliberately used.

Feelings: Hunger and Satiety

Feelings are defined as 'The mental state that accompany body states'. Feelings arise from a complex orchestration of mainly internal molecular signals involving things like hunger, satiety, thirst and pain.[7&8] Emotions are very similar but tend to be stimulated by external forces and such emotions involve fear, disgust, anger, shame, joy, admiration, envy and so on. There is of course overlap between the two. Feelings are believed to involve four stages. The first stage is the millisecond-by-millisecond monitoring of the internal biological milieu that never ceases in the human body. This endless monitoring process involves blood elements from calcium to glucose, from energy-rich molecules to blood pressure, gut motility and so on.[9] The moment that we begin to deviate from the norm, signals, known and unknown are passed to the brain, which activate a neural network response. In effect, different neurons in different parts of the brain become activated and interconnected and this constitutes the sensation of a particular feeling. The stronger the feeling, the more complex the neural map. As different neural networks are learned and memorised by the brain, our mental capacity can very rapidly align these feelings with our biological states. This has provided us with a huge evolutionary advantage by way of quick decisions in terms of behaviour in response to different biological needs. Thus the mind becomes aware of the immediate needs of the body and now moves to redress this signal. If the original monitoring system detected metabolic changes indicative of the need to replenish the body with energy, the mind detects hunger and the ensuing action is to eat. Now as nutrients enter the body, the millisecond-by-millisecond monitoring system begins to detect gradual changes in the internal metabolic processes and ultimately it now alters the known and unknown signals to the brain to indicate to the mind that satiety is being achieved. As before, the greater the degree of change in the internal signals, the more complex the neural map and thus the mind might at one level decide 'OK, I'm no longer starving' or at another level 'OK, I'm stuffed and couldn't eat another thing.' So far in this study of the regulation of food intake, there is precious little between humans and our friend the fox. So in this crucially important topic of the regulation of food intake, what distinguishes us from the fox? Why do we see fat humans but we never see a fat fox? To answer that question, we need to consider the role that the frontal cortex of the human brain plays in everyday life.

The Human Brain

No other species on earth relates to food in the way humans do. To begin with, most of us rely on someone else (farmers, food manufacturers, restaurateurs) to procure our food. We have behavioural limitations imposed on us in the form of ethics, manners, beliefs and the like. We are creatures of habit. We are incredibly social in our behaviour. We have time constraints. We have the ability to reason and understand the essential nutritional dimension of foods and how that food might impinge on our wellbeing. We experience disgust at dietary behaviours that are abnormal to our own. In effect, the biological aspect of the regulation of food intake is straightforward and logical. The behavioural aspect of food intake in humans is utterly complex and is directly under the control of the frontal cortex part of the human brain; consider the following dialogue on food choice:

Ern: What would you like for dinner, Soph?
Soph: Fresh soft shell crab, mifgash mushrooms, tigernuts and fennel.
Ern: I'm going to the local shops, not New Orleans via Jerusalem so stop fooling. What would you like to eat for dinner?
Soph: Roast lamb would be nice.
Ern: Soph, we're going to the theatre so we don't have time to roast a leg of lamb. So come on, what will I buy?
Soph: Lasagne would be fine.
Ern: Soph, we had lasagne last night which was left over from the night before. Give us a break.

75

Soph: You choose but mind my allergies.

Ern: While I'm at it, what do you want for breakfast tomorrow?

Soph: Ern, what are you at. You know my choice of breakfast, it's porridge, orange juice and tea. It always is, so why ask?

From the above we learn the following: if it isn't available, you can't eat it. The converse is also true. If it is available somebody will eat it, somewhere, someday.[10] Even if it is available, time constraints might exclude a given food choice. For certain meals, variety is paramount but for others, variety is not an option. Having lasagne for dinner three days in a row is not something Ern would accept. But Soph is clear about breakfast. It almost never changes. We also learn that food choice is *a priori* determined by health considerations, in this case allergies, but potentially involving many aspects of health including weight management. It isn't mentioned in the above, but Ern is Jewish and eats according to traditional Jewish food law. Thus besides health as a line of demarcation in food choice, we have ethnic and religious constraints. Ethical issues are involved such as those who pursue vegetarianism or veganism or are acutely conscious of fair trade issues. We don't always eat just because we are hungry but because it's the time of the day when we are expected to eat something. Price is a huge determinant of food choice and while many would like to dine on the choicest of meats, exotic mushrooms, the freshest of vegetables and so on, price is dominant.

Thus far, we have already seen that the complexity of taste, texture and flavour of foods determines each individual's food preference. And, we have just seen how the human values that are derived from our frontal cortex determine our behaviour around choosing foods and executing meals. However, these factors don't tell us much about what and how much we put on our plates, and that is the crux of the issue in the development of excess weight.

Empty Plates

Traditionally, researchers studied food choice and expected satiety using a simple scale called a visual analog scale (VAS). For example, an individual might be shown a variety of foods and asked to rate their satiating potential. They would be given a sheet with a 10 centimetre line on it, marked every centimetre starting at zero and ending at ten. The question posed might be: 'how filling do you think this food is?' where zero on the scale is 'not at all filling' and where ten on the scale is 'extremely filling'. These studies involved both pictures of foods and tastings of foods. In recent years, computer technology has allowed a new and exciting dimension to this research that will eventually supersede the VAS approach.[11] The volunteers sit in front of a computer. On the left hand side is a photograph of a standard meal (e.g. boiled potatoes). On the right hand side, pictures of varying portions of another food are shown and the subjects click on the image of that portion of the test food which equals the standard food in terms of their expectation of not feeling hungry between say lunch time and dinner time. Very large variations were found in the expectations of satiating effects of foods and the caloric serving size chosen.[12] Compared to the test meal of boiled potatoes, a serving of pasta with 200 calories was expected to yield the same level of satiety. In contrast, the satiating value of a pizza to equal that of the test meal of boiled potatoes was 385 calories. Clearly, individuals vary greatly in their expected satiety from different foods. However, two important points emerge from some of these studies. The first is that the more familiar the food the greater is the expected satiety attributes. Thus an unknown food, which might have the same dimensions and colouring as a familiar food, is likely to poorly predict satiety expectations indicating that the latter is something that is learned by individuals over time. Secondly, the expected satiety was found in several experiments to be an excellent predictor of meal size, thus performing much better than pre-meal measures of hunger or within-meal measures of fullness. As one group of reviewers put it: 'The implication is that the key opportunity to control energy intake within a meal may be the brief period of cognitive activity during portion selection, rather than during and towards the end of the meal with the onset of satiation.'[13] It would thus appear that each individual has a particular expectation of the satiating effect of foods and that each individual has a picture in their mind as to what portion of that food will meet their specific satiation needs. It is for these reasons that the title of this chapter included the words: 'the eyes have it!'

We have seen that the visual aspects of a dish or meal play a very large part in determining its gastronomic appeal. Visual aspects also influence portion size. If the portion size is too big or too small the dish will turn us off. Thus a bowl of soup the size of a large stewing pot would diminish its appeal just as a serving of soup in an egg cup would. There is a certain expectation that a bowl of soup will conform to some standard serving. If it does we are happy and our expectation is that we will finish the bowl of soup and achieve an expected level of fullness. However, we can be tricked. Researchers at Cornell University devised a study where volunteers were served a standard bowl of soup and they rated their sense of fullness.[14] A second group of volunteers were served the same soup in the same venue but this time from a bowl that was secretly connected by a tube underneath the table to a supply of soup and as the volunteers ate their soup, the soup bowl was secretly re-filled, slowly and imperceptibly. Those who ate soup from the self-filling bowl consumed 73% more than those who ate from the standard bowl. However, they did not believe they had eaten more and they did not subjectively rate themselves as feeling fuller. The visual cue of a bowl full of soup was stronger than the biological pathways regulating appetite.

This visualisation of a portion size has led some researchers to the concept of meal planning. This argument centres on the notion that unlike animals, humans have an *a priori* concept of what the portion size should be. There is some evolutionary logic to this in that the effort of preparing a meal must be rewarded by an adequate meal size but not so great that some of the food gets wasted. In general, we plan portion size such that we will subsequently either clean the plate or not be surprised by the amount of leftover food. Of course, there are occasions when we are embarrassed by the amount of food we leave behind on our plate but generally speaking, we align our selected portions to our expectations of eating all or most of the meal. Research shows that 91% of subjects reported that when they last ate a meal, they cleaned the plate.[15] This figure was 99% for breakfast, 89% for lunch and 87% for dinner. It was also higher for meals prepared at home (94%) as compared to meals eaten in a restaurant or café (79%) and it was also higher for self-selected meals (92%) as opposed to meals selected by someone else (88%). Finally, clean plates were much more common when the individual themselves chose the portion size (95%) as opposed to someone else (77%). So the vast majority of people plan to consume the entire meal at the outset and then proceed to do so. This study also showed that the main reason why people would finish the meal off even if they were full was to not waste the food.

All in all, the regulation of food intake is extraordinarily complex and whilst we share a great deal of the biological regulation of hunger and satiety with the fox and all other animals, we alone have constructed a culture which fosters the behavioural side of food choice as opposed to the biological side. However, our remarkable capacity for a truly wide variation in choice in food intake isn't necessarily learned as a youngster and following us as we grow old. We actually inherit an awful lot of food behaviour and that food behaviour is determined by internal and external cues.

Cue Appetite

It makes sense that people would plan meals in advance to provide the right amount of calories expected and to minimise waste. But as we will see in chapter eight, there is the phenomenon of 'mindless eating'. This pattern of eating isn't planned and tends to be related mainly to snacks rather than sit-down meals. To understand this pattern we need to look at the drivers of appetite, both the initiating of eating and its cessation. These 'drivers' are referred to as cues and it is held that cues are both internal (physiological) and external (environmental). Much research has been done on such cues but I choose to look back to a review published in the highly rated journal, *Science*, almost half a century ago.[16] The review was written by Stanley Schachter of Columbia University's Department of Psychology. He summarises the prevailing research with four studies covering fear, environment, time and taste. I will take each in turn.

Fear: A major effect of fear is that it considerably reduces stomach motility and stomach motility has been linked to the feeling of hunger. Earlier studies that monitored gastric motility every 15 minutes showed no differences between lean and obese subjects. The research then showed that when the stomach wasn't contracting, the feeling of hunger was identical between the lean and obese. However when the stomach contracts via gastric motility over 70% of normal subjects feel hungry while less than 50% of obese subjects feel hungry. This led Schachter to conclude that obese subjects were much less sensitive to the internal cue of gastric motility than normal weight subjects. To study this further, he devised a study with both lean and obese subjects half of whom were offered a range of different crackers with either a full or empty stomach. They were wrongly told that the experiment was about taste and that they could eat as many crackers as they liked to judge their preferences. In reality, the researchers were only interested in the amount of crackers eaten. The normal subjects ate considerably fewer crackers when their stomachs were full but for the obese, they ate the same amount of crackers whether on a prior full or prior empty stomach. Thus the obese were insensitive to the internal cue. The subjects were also connected to one of two electrical devices. The researchers explained that in one case they might encounter a minor tingling sensation (low fear) while for the other, they were told that the shocks would be painful but would do no permanent damage (high fear). No such electrical stimuli were ever given to the subjects but the implied future use of such induced two levels of fear. Again, they did the cracker test. The higher the fear factor, the fewer crackers the normal weight subjects ate but fear level had no effect on the amount of crackers the obese subjects ate. The conclusion is that internal stimuli of either a full stomach or altered stomach motility through fear had no effect on the appetite of the obese subjects. The internal stimulus is there but they cannot interpret it as they should.

Environment: Lean and obese subjects were fed on a vanilla-flavoured liquid diet for several months. Half of each group received their diet in a pitcher and they could eat as much as they liked, whenever they liked. The other half was machine fed, where they pressed a button that dispensed a mouthful of the liquid diet at each press. Both feeding systems were thus unappealing and both feeding systems were devoid of any of the normal social trappings of eating. In other words, the fun and pleasure of dining was taken away. This had no effect on the caloric intake of the normal weight subjects but the caloric intake of the obese, plummeted to well under half of the normal weight subjects and most lost weight, one woman falling from 410 pounds to 190 pounds over eight months. Here the conclusion is that the external cues for eating may be missing from the daily lives of the normal weight but their internal cues keep their weight normal. Take away the joy of eating and the obese cannot cope. They are highly reliant on external cues.

Time: Lean and obese subjects were tricked into believing that they were to take part in a physiology study where electrodes were placed on their wrists. Watches were taken from them. They entered a room at exactly 5 pm and were fitted with the electrodes, which took exactly five minutes. They were then left alone in the room with a clock on the wall for a true 30 minutes. For half the subjects, the clock ran at half the normal speed while for the other half it ran at twice the normal speed. After a true 30 minutes, the researcher returned eating crackers and offered the subjects to share them while they undid the electrodes and started a short interview. For half the subjects, the interviewer entered the room at 5.20 pm while for the other half it was 6.05 pm. Normal subjects ate more crackers when they thought it was 5.20 pm compared to when the clock read 6.05 pm. They commented that they didn't want to spoil their dinner at home snacking so close to their dinnertime. The obese subjects did the exact opposite. If it was 6.05 pm it was near dinnertime so they must be hungry so they ate more than when it was just 5.20 pm. In all instances, the true time of entry of the interviewer was 5.35 pm. This shows that normal weight subjects, truly believing the time to be 6.05 pm, can override the time external cue to control appetite. The obese cannot. The external cue 6.05 pm drives their appetite.

Taste: For this study, three groups of subjects were used, an underweight group, a normal weight group and an obese group. The subjects were offered two types of vanilla ice cream. One was a very high quality delicious smooth creamy product while the other was a bitter product. The subjects could eat as much as they liked. The obese wolfed down the high quality product, followed by a lesser amount by the normal weight subjects and even less by the underweight subjects. With the bitter product the pattern of intakes was entirely reversed but the differences were not so great. So obese people are much more sensitive to the external cue of taste compared to normal weight or underweight subjects.

All of these studies of almost 50 years ago point to a greatly altered sensitivity of obese subjects to both internal and external food cues. Fast forward by some 40 years and we can again see variation in responsiveness to internal and external cues. This study, conducted by Professor Jane Wardle and colleagues at King's College London, used two datasets, which provided cross-sectional data for two age groups of children, three to five year olds and eight to eleven year olds.[17] The advantages of using children are: (a) that childhood is a critical period for obesity development; (b) children of these ages are unlikely to manipulate their food intake to manage weight; (c) overweight and obese adults would have a long period of adiposity which itself might alter food behaviour. The parents of the children completed a child eating behaviour questionnaire and provided data on weight, height and waist circumference. A measure of 'Satiety Responsiveness – Slow Eating' (SRSE) was included in the questionnaire as was 'Enjoyment of Food' (EF). SRSE fell dramatically as body mass index or waist circumference increased and EF went in the opposite direction. Thus heavier children were more sensitive to the external cues associated with the enjoyment of food and were less likely to display sensitivity to fullness. Nothing changed in those four decades but the next step in the story, the genetic dimension to eating behaviour, will take us to another new plane. There is however one more study in this area that I want to draw on and it shows that cognitive beliefs and expectations outweigh macronutrient or energy content of a food in terms of gastronomic experiences.[18] There were four arms to the study where the same amount of calories was ingested each time and all were cherry coloured. The first two involved eating a milkshake and the second two involved eating gelatin cubes. In each of these paired studies the subjects were given a lab demonstration to explain what would happen in their gut when they ate the test meal. Treatment one involved the milkshake and the volunteers were told that on entering the stomach, the milkshake would fully dissolve in gastric acid. The test demo used water and the two dissolved into one liquid instantly. This was called the 'Liq–Liq' arm. The next groups consuming the milkshake were told that the milk would coagulate in their stomach and the relevant demo simply used cherry coloured alginate forming a big blob with a calcium chloride solution that would remain for a period in their stomach after eating the milkshake. This was the 'Sol–Liq' arm. In effect, the former elicited a sense of lack of fullness when the milkshake was eaten ('It went right through me. I'm so hungry') while the latter elicited a serious sense of fullness ('I can't remember eating anything which made me so full'). The next two arms involved eating the same quantity of calories as purple gelatin cubes, again, with two explanations as to what would happen in the gut following their ingestion. The demonstrations involved the use of hot water to indicate dissolution into gastric juice and the use of cold water to indicate a solid legacy that would eventually dissolve. Those ('Sol–Liq') that were told that the gelatin would dissolve in their stomach (the hot water demonstration) elicited responses such as 'I felt full at first but it immediately went away when the cubes turned to liquid in my stomach.' In contrast, the final group, the 'Sol–Sol' group where the gelatin cubes remained solid in cold water elicited a full feeling ('I feel like I just ate an entire buffet'). So the human sensation of satiety is very strongly associated with external suggestions. These are not 'cues' such as sight, smell or presence of food or time of day or anything like it. These demonstrations simply interfered with normal cognition, possibly forcing the respondents to think of post-ingestive events in a way they had never done so. Either way, this study shows that the human response to food intake is extraordinarily complex.

Genetics and Food Intake Patterns

In the previous chapter we saw how twin studies can play a huge role in determining body weight and in particular, excess body weight. Recent twin studies have looked at the heritability of eating behaviour.[19] Using a twin birth cohort (the Gemini cohort), Professor Wardle was able to show that in infants in the first five years of life, the heritability of appetite determinants was high when the baby eating behaviour questionnaire was applied. It was moderate for the 'Enjoyment of Food Score' (0.53) and the 'Food Responsiveness Score' (0.59). However, it was very high for the 'Slowness of Eating Score' (0.84) and the 'Satiety Responsiveness Score' (0.72). Another study used 347 twin pairs, studied first at 2.5 years of age and then again at nine years of age.[20] For two of the measures of eating behaviour ('Does not eat enough' and 'Eats too much'), there were big differences between identical and non-identical twins at 2.5 years. At nine years of age, the following measures were more highly correlated among identical twins: 'Does not eat enough', 'Eats too fast', 'Refuses to eat', 'Eats at irregular hours', 'Eats between meals' and 'Skips breakfast'. These data emphasise the important role of genetics in determining food-eating patterns. However, genetics also plays a big role in food preference, which is of course linked to the extent to which foods are found to be appetising.[21] One study with twins aged four to five years showed that the heritability of preference for foods was low for desserts, moderate for vegetables, higher still for fruits and very high for protein foods such as meat, fish and poultry. Yet another looked at neophobia in children aged eight to eleven years and found that heritability was high at 0.78.

So if twin studies tell us that food behaviour and choice have a large genetic determinant, is there any evidence to point to particular genes. The FTO gene is one possibility and the interest in this gene has been outlined in the preceding chapter with 16% of the population carrying the highest risk form of FTO with a much higher risk of obesity compared to the 46% of the population carrying the lowest risk version of the FTO gene. In one study, subjects were given a test meal with blood samples taken at regular intervals after the start of the meal and had an MRI scan of their brain to ascertain their neural response to images of high calorie foods.[22] Those with the highest risk FTO variety had greater ratings of hunger throughout the period after the meal and they also showed a very high brain response to high calorie foods. Moreover, the levels of the hormone ghrelin in their blood were much higher compared to those with the low risk FTO variety. Ghrelin is a hormone that is released from the gut to the brain to indicate the feeling of hunger. Then finally, Professor Jane Wardle's group has shown that children carrying the high risk variant of FTO show a much lower 'Food Responsiveness Score' and a much higher 'Food Enjoyment Score' with the childhood eating behaviour questionnaire.[23]

So where does all this fascinating data leave us. Firstly, it shows that appetite is the key to obesity, which may sound blindingly obvious. However, much of the research into obesity is devoted to how the main energy yielding molecules such as fat and glucose are absorbed, transported, stored, transposed and oxidised for energy. Appetite is intrinsically linked with our behavioural response to internal cues that we might share with the fox but is particularly linked to external cues, none of which bother the fox. The external cues are the man made social nature of eating and the man made organisation of the human food chain that is abundant, appetising and cheap. However, that interplay is very definitely, genetically determined. The present research landscape in nutrition is dominated by reductionist biology and by very large longitudinal studies of diet, physical activity and obesity as well as other non-communicable diseases. The future requires a shift to incorporate long-term behavioural trends into such studies and to further incorporate a greater level of brain imagining and genetic information. As to how we should individually act to optimise our weight that will be covered in later chapters. Now we turn to the other side of energy balance: physical activity.

CHAPTER EIGHT

Fitness and Fatness

The Scale of the Problem

The *Lancet* series on physical activity ('The pandemic of physical activity: global action for public health') provides a compelling case for its role in health maintenance. This series of landmark papers in this prestigious journal enumerates at length the scale of physical inactivity, its costs and its consequences.[1] For example, the average US citizen drives about 40 miles per day, half of which is for family and non-work related reasons. In 1982, the annual time spent in traffic jams was seven hours and that increased to 26 hours by 2001. Daily television viewing doubled from about four to eight hours per day between 1950 and 2000. Only 25% of the US population met the recommended physical activity levels and this had a very strong socio-economic gradient. Thus for those with less than 12 years' schooling, only 15% met the physical activity guidelines compared to 34% among those with a college education. The direct medical costs of physical inactivity are estimated at $24 billion and the overall medical costs are estimated to be $76 billion per annum. To put that into perspective, the annual budget for the FBI is just under $9 billion,[2] that of the CIA is about $44 billion[3] and the Department of Homeland Security spent just $66 billion in 2011.[4]

The global picture is just as grim. Apparently, 31% of the earth's population does not meet the minimum requirement for physical activity and according to the World Health Organization: 'The leading global risks for mortality in the world are high blood pressure (responsible for 13% of deaths globally), tobacco use (9%), high blood glucose (6%), physical inactivity (6%), and overweight and obesity (5%).'[5] Across the globe, around 5.5 million deaths could be prevented annually if physical inactivity was eliminated. Their report also states that physical inactivity accounts for 23% of all breast and colon cancers, 27% of diabetes and 30% of all cardiovascular disease.

Physical activity is the orphan of obesity. Yes, it is accepted as a factor in the epidemic of obesity by the experts but it is quickly passed over to make room for the juicier, more sensational aspects of apportioning blame to such elements of the food chain as fast food, processed food, sugar, sugar-sweetened beverages and the like. Unlike the energy intake dimension of obesity where corporate villains abound from McDonald's to Coca-Cola, there appears to be no lobby against the internet (Google), electronic (Sony) or automobile (Chrysler) giants that foster an ever-increasing sedentary lifestyle. In effect, the argument that the increasing prevalence of physical inactivity is a core cause of human obesity is often seen by the high priests of public health nutrition as an 'industry favourable' explanation and therefore would of course be eschewed by the food sector.

Food Intake or Physical Activity

The food supply explains everything according to one school of thought and one particular scientific paper is frequently cited to justify this viewpoint.[6] The study used an established quantified link between caloric intake, as measured using stable isotopes, and body weight and compared the mean body weight of US subjects in 1970 versus 2000. The differences in body weight implied a rise in caloric intake of about 500 calories a day. They then looked at what are called food disappearance data. This approach estimates the total quantity of calories produced in the US from plant and animal sources in both 1970 and 2000. The total caloric production in the US is then adjusted downwards for exports of calories and then adjusted upwards for imports of calories in foods. Finally, and crucially in this case, they adjusted for food wastage, which was estimated by the US Department of Agriculture (USDA) to be about 27%. On that basis they showed that the rise in the net supply of calories into the US market was exactly equal to the quantity of calories (500 per day) that would explain the rise in US body weight. This remains an impressive piece of work that clearly shows that the rise in US obesity has little to do with physical activity and is fully explained by the rise in the supply of calories to the US market.

About a year after that paper was published, another group of distinguished authors produced a second paper that effectively showed the total opposite: the decline in physical activity in the US over five decades could completely explain the rise in US obesity. This study drew on data documenting the pattern of US citizens employed in different industries.[7] The data showed that, for example, the percentage of persons employed in both agriculture and 'goods producing jobs' declined dramatically over the five decades from 1960 to 2010 while jobs in the service sector showed a very strong growth (from 50% to 80% of the total US jobs). In terms of goods producing jobs the decline was mainly associated with the manufacturing industry while jobs in construction and mining stayed constant. In the service sector, the growth was largely in the professional service including health and education and also in the leisure and hospitality sectors. The calories expended in a wide variety of leisure and work related activities have been carefully documented over many years where volunteers completed specific chores while wearing devices, which measured oxygen uptake per minute for each task. The uptake of oxygen can be converted into caloric requirements of tasks and the values used are known as METS (metabolic equivalent of a task). Sitting doing nothing is equal to one MET per minute while jogging at four miles per hour is six METS. Drawing on these data, the researchers were able to show that the average occupational METS fell from 2.55 to 2.30 per minute over the five decades of study. This translated into a drop in occupational expenditure of energy of 140 calories per day for men and 124 calories per day for women. The authors then used 1960 body weights and changes in caloric expenditure at work to calculate the rise in body weight that would accrue from the fall in caloric expenditure at work. Most importantly, and in contrast to the previous study, it used the most up-to-date data on US food waste.[8] Having done so they then compared their predictions of weight change to the actual rise in body weight in the US. The predicted change in body weight exactly equalled the observed weights as recorded in successive US national surveys. So here we have two studies that look at the rise in obesity in the US, one of which blames food intake and the other blames physical activity at work. The latter has the strength of taking realistic data on food loss into its model.

There are other important papers that look at the physical inactivity versus excess energy intake as causes of obesity. Two leading researchers at Cambridge's Medical Research Council Nutrition Centre published a paper with the catchy title 'Obesity in Britain: gluttony or sloth?' They showed that over the period 1950 to 1990, whereas obesity rates rose steadily (actually slightly wave-like as described earlier) caloric intake remained more or less constant. In contrast, the rise in obesity over this period was exactly matched by the rise in cars per household and hours watching television.[9]

So who is right in apportioning blame in the obesity game – physical inactivity or excess caloric intake? Whilst the scientists might argue, the general public applying common sense to their experience over the last three decades will see things quite clearly. They will have witnessed a growth in the availability of foods outside the home from fast food restaurants to high dining facilities. They will have seen food prices fall, a rise in convenience food, a rise in microwave and from-the-freezer prepared foods and in general the ubiquitous nature of the highly palatable modern food chain. By the same token they will have seen a major decline in the need for physical activity both at work and in the home. Once upon a time, offices had filing cabinets and endless files to be accessed, read and returned. It was off one's butt, a walk to the filing facility, a search, a trip back to the office and then a return trip to the filing facility. Now, the files are digitised and we don't even have to lift our backsides to work. Car assembly plants are dominated by robotic technologies and one human can now oversee what many would have had to do manually in the past. Today, the supermarket and takeaway comes to our armchairs, our commutes are now so long that for about one in five, a third of our time allocated to earning a living is in commuting on trains, buses and cars. Another indicator of how our lives have changed over time is to compare the number of steps taken per day by the average US citizen versus the average member of the Amish community, which has shunned all involvement in modern technologies in their traditional agricultural community lifestyle. On average the Amish community takes 33,000 steps per day whereas the modern non-Amish American takes just 7,300 steps per day, almost as low as a fifth of the Amish step count.[10] Clearly, the global rise in obesity has its origins in the decline of occupational physical activity and the growth of a cheap, palatable, affordable and abundant food supply.

An Epidemiological Perspective

To quantify the effects of physical activity on all-cause mortality, let us consider a recent European study that followed over 330,000 subjects for an average of 12.4 years.[11] They used an internationally accepted questionnaire to ascertain physical activity levels. Based on these data, they classified the subjects into four groups: inactive; moderately inactive; moderately active; active. Setting the mortality rate from all causes of the inactive group at 1.0, the relative reduction in such mortality fell 24% on moving into the moderately inactive group. However, there was no further benefit in moving further upwards in the activity scale. The difference in energy expenditure between the inactive and moderately inactive group was of the order of 100 calories, which equates to about a 20 minute brisk walk each day. The authors make a very significant comparison between the global mortality burden from physical inactivity and the global burden of mortality from obesity. The former is estimated at 676,000 deaths per year while the comparable figure for obesity is 337,000 deaths. Now take a minute to absorb this. The media bombards us daily with reports on obesity and health and if one mentions physical inactivity, then it is greeted as a contributory factor to obesity but nowhere near the foul and toxic effects of sugar, fast food, processed food and whatever is the latest darling of the media. Who is championing the campaign against physical inactivity? Who is shouting from the rooftops that for every death that occurs due to obesity-related illnesses, two occur from physical inactivity? The answer is of course either nobody or nuisance groups that don't understand the 'truth' about diet and obesity. But now that you know, you can be a champion of moderate physical activity as well as a champion of weight management.

As has been pointed out in chapter two, epidemiological studies can show cause and effect but intervention studies are needed to prove a true effect of physical activity on reducing obesity and obesity-related disorders. For many, physical activity means a gym and a gym means money and a commitment of some leisure time to the proposed programme. This programme will inevitably mean a mix of weights, stretching, lifting, pulling and some exercise cycling and treadmill jogging. Research shows that for 90% of fitness clubs, the attrition rate in participation is from 30 to 50%.[12] Walking on the other hand can be built into our daily lives without necessarily eating into leisure time. And walking has a profoundly beneficial effect on health. A recent analysis of intervention studies that examined the health benefits of walking shows just that. This study searched the literature for intervention studies, which began with sedentary volunteers, had a duration of at least four weeks and that always included a control group given no advice or encouragement on walking.[13] They covered 40 years of research output (1972–2012) and identified in all some 32 studies, which met all of the required entry criteria. The results on average showed: a rise in aerobic fitness which is a measure of heart and lung fitness, a decline in blood pressure, a fall in weight, body fat and BMI. Clearly, the most popular and most widely recommended form of exercise, walking, is highly effective in promoting health.

If physical activity is good and obesity is bad, then how do we combine these? In other words, how does all this risk pan out for the two extremes of lifestyle? Those who have excess body weight but who are physically active represent one extreme. Those with a perfectly normal weight but who are physically inactive represent the other. Enter the fitness–fatness debate.

The general consensus would be that all of the adverse effects of obesity, particularly high blood pressure, high blood lipids and adult onset diabetes, are reduced through physical activity. They are not eliminated, simply reduced. There are several studies worth mentioning. The first is from Finland where 18,892 men and women aged 25–74 years were followed from baseline for just under ten years.[14] At baseline, the subjects were free of all forms of heart disease and in the ensuing ten years a total of 818 cases of heart disease were recorded. When the data were controlled for all known confounding factors such as age, smoking, high blood pressure and so on, the rate of heart disease among those with moderate levels of physical activity was 30% lower compared to those who had low levels of physical activity. Those with high levels of physical activity were slightly better off with a total reduction in heart disease of about 36%. Fine, this is in line with what the preceding section, which pointed out the health benefits of physical activity. When the effects of obesity were also considered, those who were overweight had about a 20% increased risk of heart disease and among the obese, that figure rose to just under 60%. Again, that is consistent with what was met in previous chapters on the dire effects of obesity on health outcomes. Now we need to combine the data. When the two factors of physical activity and overweight were combined, setting the rate of heart disease among the lean and fit group at 1.0, the rate rose by 25% among the lean and inactive group.

Moving now to the fat but fit group, the rate was 35% higher than the control group of lean and fit. Among the group with the two downsides of obesity and physical inactivity, fat and unfit, the risk rose by 100%. As expected, the two extremes differed radically, the fit and slim versus the fat and unfit. However, there was precious little to separate out the intermediate groups, the fat and fit group and the lean and unfit group. In a similar vein, researchers at the Harvard School of Public Health completed a broadly similar study where 88,393 women aged 34 to 59 years were followed for 20 years.[15] Again, they were free of all forms of heart disease at baseline and in the follow up period there were just fewer than 1,500 cases of non-fatal heart disease and just under 900 cases of fatal heart disease. In this instance, fatness was measured using the ratio of waist to hip, a measure of abdominal obesity. Again, the best scenario was to be slim and fit and the worst was to be fat and unfit. However, there was very little difference between those who were at the top level of fatness and fitness versus those that were at the lowest level of fatness and fitness. Finally, we can consider a meta-analysis of all known studies, which examined the mortality risk of the fit and fat groups versus all others.[16] The researchers set out minimum criteria for a study to be considered. Firstly, the studies had to be longitudinal, that is, a group of healthy people recruited at baseline and then followed for several years (average of 11.4 years), the study had to include objective measures of cardiorespiratory fitness and had to have records of BMI. Of the 66 studies, which showed potential interest after the initial screen, only ten studies met the strict inclusion criteria. Let's first compare the mortality rate of the unfit groups. There was a two-fold higher risk of mortality among the unfit normal weight or unfit overweight groups compared to the ideal of fit and slim. That figure for the obese and unfit group grew to a three-fold higher risk. Now we can compare the ideal slim and fit group with the fit and overweight and fit and obese groups. The risk of mortality in these fat and fit groups did not differ statistically from the ideal group. So, if you take a look at your lifestyle and deem yourself to be overweight or sedentary, my strong advice would be to first tackle the sedentary side and to take up walking, preferably integrated as much as possible into your daily routine. This is something that will be addressed in greater detail when we come to weight loss strategies.

What are the Physical Recommendations?

The next question to be addressed is what types of physical activity, and at what intensity, is needed to obtain the benefits of being fit. This has been addressed in a US report, which issued guidelines for physical activity for children, adults and older adults.[17] Their advice for adults is thus:

- All adults should avoid inactivity. Some physical activity is better than none, and adults who participate in any amount of physical activity gain some health benefits.
- For substantial health benefits, adults should do at least 150 minutes (2 hours and 30 minutes) a week of moderate-intensity, or 75 minutes (1 hour and 15 minutes) a week of vigorous-intensity aerobic physical activity, or an equivalent combination of moderate- and vigorous-intensity aerobic activity. Aerobic activity should be performed in episodes of at least 10 minutes, and preferably, it should be spread throughout the week.
- For additional and more extensive health benefits, adults should increase their aerobic physical activity to 300 minutes (5 hours) a week of moderate-intensity, or 150 minutes a week of vigorous-intensity aerobic physical activity,

or an equivalent combination of moderate- and vigorous-intensity activity. Additional health benefits are gained by engaging in physical activity beyond this amount.

• Adults should also do muscle-strengthening activities that are moderate or high intensity and involve all major muscle groups on 2 or more days a week, as these activities provide additional health benefits.

The bottom line is simple. Doing some physical activity as opposed to none is a start. Being active for 30 minutes per day for five days of the week will bring most of the benefits of physical activity.

Welcoming the Smart Office

Walking, along with other recreational activities such as golf, tennis, football, jogging, swimming and so on are all forms of energy expenditure associated with physical activity. What characterises these is that they are all volitional. One chooses to play golf or go swimming, walking, jogging cycling or whatever over other options for spending one's time. But there is another form of physical activity, which is not volitional and this is referred to as non-exercise activity thermogenesis (NEAT). NEAT has often been referred to in the literature as 'fidgeting' but it is a little more than that.[18] For example, if you go for a walk at lunch time that is volitional exercise, but if you leave your office to visit a colleague down the corridor to discuss some topic then that involves NEAT. NEAT operates in the home as housework, house repair, gardening, car maintenance, collecting the kids or grandkids from school and other activities, shopping, going to games, to church and so on. In work, it is the physical exertion of a shop assistant standing, fetching, carrying, re-sorting, packing, smiling or the physical exertion of a company executive sitting at the desk, walking to meetings in the building, standing giving a presentation, talking on the phone, lifting books or files to and from shelves, walking to lunch, making tea or coffee, making a sandwich, and so forth.

The pioneer of NEAT or 'fidgeting' is Professor James Levine, an endocrinologist from the Mayo clinic. The first of his studies to consider is one that set out to quantify exactly how many calories were expended in the minimal movement seen in a typical modern day office.[19] Some 24 healthy subjects agreed to take part. The first measurement made was to estimate resting metabolic rate and thus they lay motionless for one hour while breathing into a device that can indirectly measure caloric expenditure. That gave an average value of 620 calories per eight hours. This resting metabolic rate is simply a reference point. Next we move to four levels of activity as set out below:

Activity for seven hours per working day	Calories expended over seven hours	Assume one hour walking at one mile per hour	Total eight-hour caloric expenditure
Sitting motionless	562	196	758
Sitting while fidgeting (free movement of arms, legs, torso, head)	822	196	1,018
Standing motionless	612	196	808
Standing with permission to emulate, at their discretion, activities typical of an office day	1,033	196	1,229

In effect, just sitting almost all day at your desk with 60 minutes of strolling about to chat or going to meetings or whatever, accounts for 758 calories per working day. If an individual were to use a standing desk and also engage in one hour of sauntering around the building, then an extra 471 calories per working day would be burned off. Even if standing all day was too much and the day was split evenly between sitting and fidgeting and standing and fidgeting, the difference would be 260 calories. An extra 260 or so calories expended every day without any increase in energy intake would see weight fall and if energy intake increased to meet this 300 calories, then energy balance would be maintained. It is thus crystal clear that if we could adjust our office lifestyle with some smart designs and incentives, then we could make inroads into combating physical inactivity and obesity.

Professor Levine then makes an obvious point: 'If 47% of US citizens do not achieve the minimum target for physical activity and if 23% of Americans are totally sedentary with no volitional exercise, then clearly, NEAT becomes a major player in overall energy expenditure.' To test this Levine recruited 16 non-obese subjects and measured their exact energy needs using an indirect calorimeter.[20] Once he had established their energy needs, he fed the volunteers 1,000 extra calories per day over eight weeks above their calculated requirements. The volunteers had at baseline a maximum of two sessions of physical activity per week and they had to strictly adhere to that baseline level of physical activity. All food was provided by the research team and very carefully apportioned to get an extra 1,000 calories per day for the eight-week period. Energy expenditure was made using a very advanced technique involving stable isotopes of water that is generally regarded as the Rolls-Royce of the measurement and every bit as expensive. Over the eight-week period, the average gain in body fat, as measured by another very sophisticated X-ray technique (DEXA Scan) was 389 grams with a range of 56 to 687 grams. Because the volunteers got bigger during the study, their resting metabolic rate got bigger by 79 calories per day. Now it is critical to remember that in this study, there was no change in volitional exercise since this was stringently controlled at the low levels seen at baseline. Thus, any changes in energy expenditure not explained by resting metabolic rate or the thermic effects of food, had to do with changes in NEAT since volitional exercise was held constant. Thus when the authors looked to see what aspect of energy expenditure correlated with the gain of body fat over the eight weeks, neither the basal metabolic rate or the thermic effect of food were in any way capable of explaining this gain in fat. But activity thermogenesis did, and almost in a perfectly straight line. The lowest gains of body fat following eight weeks of overfeeding to the level of 1,000 calories per day were strongly associated with higher levels of activity thermogenesis which can be attributed to NEAT. If we were to extrapolate from this highly controlled experiment to the real world we can see an abundance of putatively cheap, energy dense and highly palatable foods tending to drive caloric intake upwards and we can also see that those that are active in everyday life efforts other than volitional sport, are well capable of maintaining energy balance. But just as the so-called cheap, palatable and energy dense foods are ubiquitous in society, so too is the sedentary promoting environment.

Thus the final challenge to James Levine was to do the real experiment. A group of 36 volunteers agreed to swap their normal sitting desk to one which could also operate as a treadmill with the flick of a switch. This was to alter the physical environment of work to increase NEAT and to see if it actually improved NEAT and energy balance.[21] The volunteers held sedentary jobs at a financial services company and they agreed to exchange their traditional desk for a treadmill desk which could act (a) as a normal desk, (b) a standing desk and (c) a standing desk with a treadmill underneath with a maximum rate of walking of two miles per hour. A wide range of measurements was made and daily activities were recorded using a fancy step meter known as an accelerometer. By the end of the year, daily activity units increased 25% and body weight fell by 1.4 kilograms on average, and up to 2.3 kilograms among those who were obese at the outset. Systolic blood pressure also fell by four units of mercury.

Clearly, it is possible to alter the built environment at the workplace to increase physical activity and to better manage body weight.

Physical activity is still the orphan of energy balance but the scale of evidence is so great that sooner or later it will be at least on a par with obesity. To get there will be a struggle. Firstly, diet-related energy balance is owned by the media and together with the corridors of power a most attractive array of guilty corporations and 'toxic' foods are the primary anti-obesity targets. Secondly, this group does all in its power to see the promotion of physical activity as a real but not a priority problem and as a distraction to the real issue of diet and energy balance and a cause fostered by the food industry in its defence.

Before moving to the latter part of this book, we need to take one final look at some potential contributors to weight gain. These are frequently covered in the news media and all have a high scientific dimension. The list is by no means exhaustive, just illustrative.

CHAPTER NINE

A Miscellany of Matters

The media loves a story and a good story teller so a group of scientists who have some wow-factor research will always be welcome and the more serious the subject, and the more heavy hitters backing it, the more likely it is to rise from tabloid headlines to serious inside reading even making it to the exalted week-end magazine section. But for every scientific story that scores on the wow scale of the popular media, there are stories that frankly are too boring for the media. In the fields of diet, physical inactivity and obesity, many such wow and boring stories abound, and in this chapter I have selected just a few to try and cast some scientific light on their contribution to the problem at hand or its resolution.

The Maternal Role

Throughout this book I have referred to the fact that unlike the fox, human infants are soft-wired to account for the accidents of birthplace, inherited religion, language, cuisine, table manners, folk tradition – sung, spoken and danced – and by all its wide cultural influences and needs. The fox cub and the baby inherit their maternal and paternal gene sequences at conception and these will never change in sequence. But genetic material is made up of long sequences of material called genes and some of these are adjusted during early development to, so to speak, sing louder or softer than would be the case for nearby genes or by the very same genes in other animals. At a simple basis, all genetic material is always found in all cells much to the crime scene investigator's delight. Any trace of human tissue will have the full genetic code. But the ear does not have the gene to smell, or the nose that to hear, or the arm to remember your name. Cells keep the relevant genetic material needed for the organ's function in tip top shape but unimportant genes are silenced, put to sleep so to speak. This is the process of up-regulating or down-regulating genes. In the nose, the genes for smell are up-regulated while those of taste are down-regulated. It is the opposite to the tongue. During human development we refer to the first 1,000 days that are equivalent to the period of pregnancy (280 days) and the first two years of life (730 days). During this period, unlike the fox, the mother and in particular the infant are referred to as in a plastic state as to future development. If times are hard, nutritionally speaking, that is one message and that sets the expression of all the metabolic genes in one direction. If times are good, nutritionally speaking, the metabolic genes are expressed at a different level. The genes thus set, are set for life. Expectation is built into our biological master plans. The best explanation of this critical period of life *in utero* is the BBC documentary: 'The Nine Months that Made You.'[1]

Maternal nutrition only plays a role in offspring wellbeing if she is pregnant. But the exact timing of that undernutrition and its severity profoundly influences that setting of the master plan of life and that master plan, if there is a mismatch to its expectation, can leave to adult diseases of all organs studied to date, and that includes obesity-related conditions. Of course, it multiplies, when obese women have obese babies who are at a far higher risk of developing obesity than those born of leaner mums. All in all, ignoring the vast literature on this topic in our learned libraries is at our peril. It remains a fact that looking after the nutritional wellbeing of young adults of childbearing age must be a public health priority. But that doesn't hit the activists' radar, as I will outline in the last chapter.

Our Human Rat Race

The poor have indeed always been with us. The US government estimates that food insecurity in 2013 affected about one in seven families and that severe food insecurity affected one in twenty households.[2] The FAO definition of food insecurity is: 'A situation that exists when people lack secure access to sufficient amounts of safe and nutritious food for normal growth and development and an active and healthy life.' There are two consequences to this nutrition poverty trap. The first is that real indices of poor nutritional status emerge, simply from inadequate food intake. Thus in the US, among women who are from food insecure families, they are several times more likely to suffer iron deficiency anaemia based on actual blood measurements.[3] This is found for many other micronutrients in the US literature and is also reflected globally.[4] Poverty provokes malnutrition. The second consequence of poverty is poor food choice.

This may be partly based on level of education but it is also due to a food chain where more nutritious foods are more expensive and where affordable foods have very high energy densities per unit price, leading to obesity. To that end Professor Adam Drewnowski and his colleagues at the University of Washington conducted a systematic review and analysis of the contribution of food prices and diet cost to socio-economic disparities in diet quality and health.[5] The authors conclude: 'socioeconomic disparities in diet quality may be explained by the higher cost of healthy diets. Identifying food patterns that are nutrient rich, affordable, and appealing should be a priority to fight social inequalities in nutrition and health.' However, when we begin to consider the lower quantity of nutrient intakes among the socially disadvantaged, we must also remember that it is among this group that we have lower levels of schooling, poorer housing, more unemployed, more crime, more drug abuse, more depression, more suicide and more desperation. It is tough being poor. Moreover, we need to also return to the role of happiness I alluded to earlier in the pursuit of healthy eating. If we have to tick one box only, which would you prefer?

Box 1: The child is now going to school regularly, seems to be enjoying it and is pretty damn smarter than anyone thought with constantly good grades. The child still eats a diet that could be much improved.

Box 2: The child is now taking a cereal breakfast with chocolate flavoured milk and is eating a lot less fast food and soda. The child has little or no interest in school.

You pick, but my guess would be that the vast majority would pick from Box 1. Again and again I say to those writing top down health eating manifestos: your audience is not a clean slate. It is mightily muddied with a multitude of problems, fears, biases and phobias. Poverty has always been with us but now the price of the food chain has fallen dramatically such that the poor can now afford to get obese. But today's society does not leave the middle to upper classes without their problems.

Jay Rayner, a celebrated UK food critic, journalist, broadcaster and writer has described shopping experiences in the 1960s in his excellent book: *A Greedy Man in a Hungry World.*[6] His mother would queue and pay for butter in one area of Sainsbury's supermarket, then do the same for meat and so on for whatever else she wanted. Food shopping took a morning and rightly, women began to look at this as an impediment to their right to hold down a job. But Rayner points out that in 1962 average annual pay in the UK was £799, which rose to £26,200 in 2012 (a 33-fold increase). However, the respective cost of an average house rose from £2,670 to £245,000 in the same period (a 92-fold increase). Now a job for both spouses became a necessity, not just a right. The result is that from six months onwards, about 12 hours a day of a toddler's life are in someone else's hands other than the parents (crèches, pre-schools, carers, grand-parents) and that includes a significant part of food choice and overall toddler food management.

Of the modern world, in the context of studying it in regards to obesity and physical inactivity, it should be noted that:

- Most families work to help pay the rising mortgages that might these days be in negative equity and most strive hard to make family life a happy life. That might involve some instilling of health eating patterns but it will also involve the pursuit of affordable family happiness through treats including meals outside the home where frankly rules are greatly relaxed.
- One in five EU citizens is engaged in shift work with an obvious impact on eating habits and sharing meals with families.[7]
- Results from this meta-analyses based on these available data showed that night shift work was significantly associated with an increased risk of obesity (66%), high blood glucose and high blood pressure (both at 30%).

Clearly, we have constructed a society that has been mega-successful in sending people to outer space, that lives in a digital highway with instant access to all and sundry, good or bad, and with endless wondrous achievements and sadly, some terrible records of inhumanity. And when we whittle all our problems down to diet and health, a lot of the causes come hand in hand with the design of social behaviour that give us intercontinental nuclear devices, the Olympic Games and the automobile. You can live like the Maasai and weigh like the Maasai or live like the Yanks and weigh like the Yanks. Researchers have articulated the case that affluence has not always brought happiness. It changes our lives but not always in a happier direction. Today we demand instant pleasures, not ones based on long-term planning and personal sacrifice.[8] We are exposed to a bewildering flow of technological novelty, which can be disorientating and alienating. Our overall trust is diminished by the constant flow of ads championing ever new innovations. They go on to show that as we have become more affluent, we have become less satisfied with life using a multi-approach measure of psychological satisfaction. Why should we expect food habits to be unaffected by such developments?

The Human Microbiome – Your Gut Bacteria

When I was a graduate student at the University of Sydney Veterinary School (the early 1970s), human nutrition texts regarded what we call fibre today as 'roughage', a component of the diet, which those in human nutrition at the time regarded as bothersome, especially for people with tender guts. Indeed, low roughage diets were recommended for constipation, the complete opposite of today. It was a fellow countryman of mine, Dr Denis Burkitt, working in East Africa who is credited with the revival of dietary fibre as an essential component of health, most importantly, gut health.[9] Of course, in time, the inevitable followed and we had the F-Plan Diet, a high fibre diet to help weight loss.

Fibre, from a chemical point of view, represents a form of plant-based dietary carbohydrate that humans cannot digest and so passes on through the small intestine until it reaches the large intestine, where it is fermented by our gut bacteria in an oxygen-free environment. Whereas the rest of the human body oxidises carbohydrate in an oxygen-rich environment to yield carbon dioxide, water and energy, the gut microflora only take this oxidation half way to produce very short chain fats and energy. The bugs take the energy and most of the short chain fats enter our blood stream where some are then burned properly for energy, carbon dioxide and water and others are used to make all sorts of biological chemicals.

The next phase of dietary fibre and colonic flora research saw the emergence of the tools of molecular biology that allowed scientists for the first time to characterise with precision the exact balance of different types of bacteria in the human microbiome as it was now referred to. As with many other instances, the new technology led to an explosion in interest in the microbiome (the new name for the gut microflora) and health and with it, regrettably, a lot of unsubstantiated speculation. In the case of obesity there are some excellent data that tend to show how the human microbiome can contribute to obesity. The big question is to quantify this effect. Sometimes one can hear presentations that talk of the role of the gut microflora in extracting the last scintilla of energy from plant non-digestible carbohydrates and that this final extraction of energy from food can tip the balance toward obesity. In some instance the speakers will talk of people who eat 60 g/d of dietary fibre. In Ireland, probably typical of the northern EU, the mean fibre intake is 19 g/d and the top 5% of fibre consumers are at 34 g/d.[10] This is a long way off the oft-cited figure of 60 g/d. In reality, fibre at its present level of consumption accounts for about 30 calories per day or 1% of caloric intake. Fibre intakes are generally inadequate for proper gastrointestinal function so we should probably increase our fibre intake by say 6 g/d. At most this would add about 10 calories per day. Thus the argument that fibre contributes to obesity by extracting energy from food via the microbiome is not really worth bothering about at this stage. It should also be noted, that the mega fashion of the human microbiome in human biology extends well beyond obesity. A quick look at the following diseases linked to microbiome shows an enormous level of interest across many areas (number of published papers in brackets): at the high end we have cancer (105), diabetes (688), allergy (682), irritable bowel syndrome (n=245) and liver disease (n=118) and at the lower end we have gum disease (n=192), autism (n=84), hyperactivity (n=6), baldness (n=4) and dandruff (n=3). Something that science seeks to implicate so widely in the disease spectrum must carry a lot of serious doubt. That won't help those trying to seriously reveal the true role of the human microbiome in obesity.

The second area where the microbiome is argued to contribute to obesity is via the various signals that the microbiome secretes and which may contribute to the metabolic mechanisms of obesity. The evidence comes from two main areas. One is the use of mice that are bred from birth in a germ free environment.[11] Thus they have no microbiome and in fact they fail to get obese on diets that normally make mice fat. However, when they are treated with faeces from a normal mice microbiome and then removed from the highly sterile germ free facilities, they quickly develop obesity. That of course is meaningless to the human situation since we are never germ free although several scientists often allude to the increased levels of obesity and the growth in the use of antibiotics. Again, this is a weak area. Finally, scientists have looked at indicators of the composition of the human microbiome and how this changes with weight loss and weight gain. Yes there are changes, which correlate weight and the composition of the microbiome. But what is driving what? Is the microbiome driving the weight or is the weight driving the microbiome?

Finally, this area has received quite a critical review entitled 'Microbiome science needs a healthy dose of scepticism' in the prestigious journal, *Nature*.[12] The author's first point of criticism is that the techniques used to characterise the microbiota genome often lack direct links to known functions. He points out that his team has shown that vaccination eliminated 30% of known pneumococcal strains in a human population but only because they knew which genes to focus on. In the case of the human microbiota genome, we might know that it differs between say, normal weight and obese subjects. But that's all we know. We cannot tell what part of the microbiota genome is directly linked in a causal manner to obesity. His second criticism is linked to this in that cause and effect are misinterpreted when looking at gut microbiota. He cites a paper, which shows that changes in the human microbiota correlate with measures of frailty in older persons. So too did dietary patterns. The conclusion was that poor diet altered the gut microbiota and thus led to frailty. The opposite was not considered, namely, that frailty led to poor diets that in turn altered gut microbiome patterns. His third criticism is that most of the studies lack any mechanistic explanation based on experimental investigation. In that respect the field is similar to nutritional epidemiology where correlations dominate and shape policy in the absence of any experimental proof. So if we consider the microbiome-diet-frailty issue, a simple test would be to take a cohort of frail persons and through physiotherapy, counselling and nutritional support reduce their frailty. If a significant improvement in frailty had no effect on the microbiome, we can dismiss that theory. Alternatively, frail persons could receive faecal transplants to modify their microbiota and examine the effect of improved microbiota on frailty. Those studies, which are very realistic, would answer the true cause and effect question here but they are never done.

His fourth criticism relates to the quality of the data on the microbiota and health vis-à-vis the real world. He highlights the fact that many of the studies that show the importance of the gut microbiota are conducted in germ-free mice. Such mice live in an aseptic bubble that makes them generally ill and with poor food intake. Finally he asks if there might be a confounding factor such that the real force driving the disease is one thing and the altered micro-biota simply an observer, equally affected by the true driver. Indeed, twin studies show that our genetic makeup plays a major part in shaping our gut microbiome composition. Certain groups of specific bacteria are highly inheri-table and these specific bacterial groups are also associated with the heritability of a normal weight range. For my own part, I have an open but critical mind in relation to the microbiota and despite its present high end fashion in biological sciences, I remain unconvinced that the gut microbiome is a major driver of obesity. It may contribute to some as yet unknown aspect but it cannot explain the modern epidemic of obesity. It goes without saying that when it comes to gut health in its strictest definitions, the human microbiome plays a huge role in a healthy gut just as we believed from the early days of Denis Burkitt.

Food Addiction

Among the stigmas allotted to the obese is that of an inability to manage and control food intake. It is an attribute, which as we will see, complements many other such attributes of the obese from lack of self-control to laziness to weakness. As the role of the brain in the regulation of food intake evolved, many began to attribute a disorder of brain function as a basis for human obesity and thus the concept of food addiction emerged. At first, this was an area of serious academic research and while that may still be the case, it has been overshadowed by the public perception that indeed certain foods are addictive to certain people and among the obese; food addiction is a major problem. It is a view stoked by the popular print and electronic media. Because of its widespread entry into the food–weight issue, it is important to take time to ask hard questions of the evidence.

We can start with known addictive substances and seek to understand what they have in common in inducing a state of addiction. According to the American Society of Addictive Medicine, the following characteristics and definitions of addiction apply:

> Addiction is a primary, chronic disease of brain reward, motivation, memory and related circuitry. Dysfunction in these circuits leads to characteristic biological, psychological, social and spiritual manifestations. This is reflected in an individual pathologically pursuing reward and/or relief by substance use and other behaviors.

> Addiction is characterized by inability to consistently abstain, impairment in behavioral control, craving, diminished recognition of significant problems with one's behaviors and interpersonal relationships, and a dysfunctional emotional response. Like other chronic diseases, addiction often involves cycles of relapse and remission. Without treatment or engagement in recovery activities, addiction is progressive and can result in disability or premature death.

Clearly, the medical treatment of addiction recognises the central role of the brain in the reward an addict receives from substance abuse. It also paints the typical picture we associate with addiction namely an unrelenting craving for the addictive substance, which dominates all social and emotive aspects of the addict's life. The exact and defining clinical criteria of addiction can be found in the recently published *Diagnostic and Statistical Manual of Mental Disorders*, version 5 (*DSM-5*).[13] The *DSM-5* defines a 'substance use disorder' as the presence of at least two of eleven criteria, which are clustered in four groups:

1. Impaired control: (1) taking more or for longer than intended, (2) unsuccessful efforts to stop or cut down use, (3) spending a great deal of time obtaining, using, or recovering from use, (4) craving for substance.

2. Social impairment: (5) failure to fulfill major obligations due to use, (6) continued use despite problems caused or exacerbated by use, (7) important activities given up or reduced because of substance use.

3. Risky use: (8) recurrent use in hazardous situations, (9) continued use despite physical or psychological problems that are caused or exacerbated by substance use.

4. Pharmacologic dependence: (10) tolerance to effects of the substance, (11) withdrawal symptoms when not using or using less.

Against that background, let us consider some of these aspects in relation to food. The first must involve the brain's reward system. This system involves a neurotransmitter called dopamine, which is released from one part of the brain and taken up by others leading to a heightened sense of pleasure. The generation of such pleasure is central to many basic survival instincts such as eating, sex and social interaction and such heightened pleasure responses helped drive a successful evolutionary trajectory. High fat, and particularly high sugar foods, elicit a strong dopamine release outcome sufficient nonetheless to foster the concept that sugary foods are addictive along the lines of well-established legal and illegal substances of abuse.[14] Whilst this line of thought might seem logical and attractive, there are alternative views to be considered.[15]

The human brain, as we have seen, is an obligate glucose user. In other words on a typical day-to-day basis, the brain only uses glucose as a fuel. Muscles and other tissues can also use glucose but they are also big users of fat for energy. Not so the brain. For a neonate, about 75% of all calories go to the brain. Quite simply, the fox is born hard-wired and has almost nothing to learn as a newborn cub. A newborn baby has to learn the language, culture, manners, ethics and overall social norms that apply to the community into which it is born. That cannot be hard-wired and thus the brain is on overdrive in infancy. This high dependency on calories continues up to the sixth month where 66% of calories are used by the brain falling to 50% at two years, 33% at ten years and remaining static in adulthood at 25% of all calories consumed.[16] Now if the brain is so demanding of calories and specifically so demanding of glucose calories, could the dopamine pleasure response to glucose ingestion not simply be a survival reaction, a response which says: 'Well done, this is just what I need.' Indeed, artificial sweeteners, which do not release any glucose into the blood stream, elicit a strong dopamine response. So, perhaps, the sensation of sweetness elicits an expectation of an immediate and rapid delivery to the brain of its highly preferred fuel, glucose.[17] So, the first thing we can say about sugar and food addiction is that sugar does stimulate a significant release of dopamine as do addictive drugs and alcohol, but that it remains not impossible that this is actually an evolutionary positive feedback derived from the brain's utter insistence on the use of glucose as a fuel.

The final issue to be considered is the addictive substance. It is generally regarded, by those upholding the food addiction hypothesis, that this addictive substance is sugar, specifically sucrose. As has already been pointed out, there are ample data to show that obesity rates are not driven by sugar specifically but by all calories and all energy sources. Moreover, we will see that weight loss is entirely dependent on a caloric deficit irrespective of the sources of this caloric deficit. So linking sugar per se uniquely to obesity is fraught with challenges. And then there is the question of evidence that sucrose meets all the needs of a typical substance of abuse. What evidence is there that increasing amounts of sugar are needed to satisfy the addiction? What data exists to link obesity with any putative withdrawal symptoms from a denial of access to sugar? What data exists to show that sugar consumption among putative addicts to sugar interferes with essential activities of daily life? Do such people continue to gorge on sugar, knowing that sugar is uniquely 'responsible' for their obesity? The answer to all these questions is that no such data exists and what does exist is both contradictory and sparse.

In an attempt to bypass the restrictive criteria of the *DSM-5* definitions of addiction, researchers at Yale have developed the Yale Food Addiction Score (YFAS),[18] which brings me to the second study that used the Yale Food Addiction Score.[19] Most criteria to measure addiction are based on clinical models but the Yale version is specifically designed to examine the hypothesis of food (fat and sugar) addiction. The researchers conducted a weight loss intervention study in 178 severely obese subjects (mean BMI of 36.1 kg/m²) in a weight loss programme, which used behavioural therapy to reduce body weight over a six-month period. They hypothesised that those patients that showed signs of food addiction according to YFAS would be the least successful in weight loss and that significantly more of those with food addiction would drop out. Both hypotheses were shown not to be valid. There was no difference in weight loss between the two groups and there was no difference in attrition. This is by far the largest study to examine food addiction in relation to weight loss.

Consider a study in which alcoholics and social drinkers are compared for their ability to abstain from alcohol or to minimise their alcohol intake. The predicted outcome would be that the alcoholics would fare much worse because their addiction to alcohol is so strong. But that doesn't happen with this measure of food addiction. In all, some 15% of subjects were declared food addictive at baseline which tallies with the general range seen among the obese population seeking treatment (15–20%). Their 'addiction' to food as measured by the Yale scale is so weak that it is simply over-ridden by a behavioural therapy programme. All in all, while the concept of food addiction might seem attractive, the biology just doesn't stack up. But, in the area of public health nutrition, why let the facts spoil a good media story!

Forget the Gym – Take up the Knife

It is the norm to manage diet-related diseases with clinical management, mostly through dietary and physical activity, counselling, and also through drugs for diabetes, high blood pressure and elevated cholesterol. If someone weighs 80 kilograms and wants to lose 5 kilograms, that is achievable by most accounts – difficult and challenging – but achievable over time. If someone weighs 130 kilograms and wants to lose 35 kilograms, then that is a truly mighty challenge. Since we know how high the relapse rate is in weight loss, as high as 90% in unsupervised loss and 50% in supervised weight management, then one can reasonably ask: 'What's the point?' Don't bother wasting time on how the weight was gained the question is what do we do? If we do nothing, things will deteriorate, particularly diabetes, osteoarthritis, depression, etc. So what's to be done? Well surgical management of obesity remains an option but it is still seen as a drastic risk laden and somewhat unnatural way to tackle what we deem to be a disease of lifestyle. Strangely, we surrender to the orthopaedic surgeon to manage common knee and hip problems, to the cardiac surgeon for pacemakers, stents and at the last resort transplants, and to the plastic surgeon for droops, bulges, wrinkles and the like. So why not give the surgical option its day in court?

Unlike medical or nutritional therapy, double blind, randomised, crossover, placebo-controlled or Rolls-Royce studies are impossible. Someday some surgeon innovates as a last ditch effort and discovers a new technique, obviously having tried it out first on animal models. Others follow and a body of knowledge is built up. But it won't involve the Rolls Royce of clinical medicine for obvious ethical reasons. At present, that body of evidence favours surgical management of obesity when it has reached fairly severe conditions. If the severity is left to linger on for too long, irreparable damage might be done to organs such as the pancreas. I will take one study, a Swedish obesity study, published in *The New England Journal of Medicine*, to make a basic point about efficacy and then I'll look at cost effectiveness. There were two groups, one on whom gastric (bariatric) surgery was performed to treat obesity and another, broadly matched, was treated with usual dietary and lifestyle intervention.[20] Some managed this on their own and some had professional help. The groups were large, 1,658 and 1,771 respectively and the follow up period was long-term at 15 years. Type 2 diabetes was the primary outcome. Whereas at baseline, no cases of diabetes were noted in either group, the control group reached a level of diabetes of 28.4 cases per 1,000 persons while in the surgically managed group, the level was 6.8 cases per 1,000, a more than four-fold difference. Weight loss hit 30 kilograms in the surgical group at year one but this levelled off to 20 kilograms by year eight, remaining constant thereafter. There was no weight loss in the control group irrespective of whether they managed their efforts at weight loss, alone or with professional help.

From an economic point of view, US data suggest that keyhole bariatric surgery costs $17,000 while open bariatric surgery costs $26,000.[21] Based on a study of 3,651 patients who underwent surgery for obesity compared to matched controls who did not, the insurance companies recouped their full costs after two years with keyhole surgery and four years after open surgery. Thus from year three on, those who had keyhole surgery were 'in profit' so to speak, that is at zero cost to the health insurer.

The points raised in this chapter are intended to finish off an overview of the factors that drive obesity in our lives. Now we need turn to its management; but first we need to firmly grasp and respect the psychiatric conditions that forever accompany the curse of global obesity.

CHAPTER TEN

Obesity: The Fears and the Phobias

Obesity is always 'slammed' by the media and the participating activists. It is bad, ugly and a serious failure on a generation that thrives on incredibly successful achievements from electronics, to transport, to drug therapy, to air travel and the like. Frankly, it is an embarrassment to modern society and it has, whether we like it or not, shaped our tolerance of the problem. In this short chapter, I want to delve into this sad and depressing world view.

Stigmatisation of Fat

Few anecdotes on the stigmatisation of obesity matter more than that of Gina Score. Her account is outlined in grim detail below:

> One anecdote reported by National Public Radio is that of Gina Score, a 14-year-old girl in South Dakota sent in the summer of 1999 to a state juvenile-detention camp. Gina was characterized as sensitive and intelligent, wrote poetry, and was planning to skip a grade when she returned to school. She was sent to the facility for petty theft—stealing money from her parents and from lockers at school 'to buy food'. She was said to have stolen 'a few dollars here, a few dollars there' and paid most of the money back. The camp, run by a former Marine and modeled on the military, aimed, in the words of an instruction manual, to 'overwhelm them with fear and anxiety'. On July 21, a hot humid day, Gina was forced to begin a 2.7-mile run/walk. Gina was 5 feet 4 inches tall, weighed 224 pounds, and was unable to complete even simple physical exercises such as leg lifts. She fell behind early but was prodded and cajoled by instructors. A short time later, she collapsed on the ground panting, with pale skin and purple lips. She was babbling incoherently and frothing from the mouth, with her eyes rolled back in her head. The drill instructors sat nearby

drinking sodas, laughing, and chatting, accusing Gina of faking, within 100 feet of an air-conditioned building. After 4 hours with Gina lying prostrate in the sun, a doctor came by and summoned an ambulance immediately. Gina's organs had failed and she died.[1]

I was recently at a self-service restaurant in an international airport, when a member of our group, a nutritionist, female, tall and quite skinny, slammed down her tray, muttering under her breath. When asked what bothered her, she commented thus: 'That stupid fat woman, with layers of chips and other fatty foods and of course the token can of diet soda, spent an age rummaging in her bloody untidy bag for her purse and then proceeded to sift through endless coins to pay her flaming bill. So annoying was that fat woman.' Spoken like a true bigot. My colleague hit on several of the typical fat bigot buttons. The fat lady was stupid, she ate badly, she was untidy and altogether she was not very with it, as they say. At no stage did my colleague note that because the lady was fat she had a higher than average energy requirement and thus needed more food to maintain her weight. It didn't dawn on my colleague that the lady in question might have spent a week in the company of someone as intolerant as my friend and was delighted to be free to let it all hang loose at the airport. Maybe she was embarking on a sad trip or maybe she didn't like flying and also maybe she lived in a jurisdiction with a different currency and wanted to get rid of as much change as possible. No, my friend operated a System 1 mindless knee-jerk reaction to the fat lady. Her reaction is absolutely ubiquitous in society. To set the context, let's first consider how children see the overweight and obese.

Just over 50 years ago, a study was published, exploring the attitudes of schoolchildren to obesity. The study was repeated with exactly the same protocol in 2003. Almost 500 US children in their fifth and sixth grades took part with about half of the sample from a wealthy suburb of New Jersey and the other half from a poorer suburb.[2] The children were shown six drawings of children where the drawings illustrated children of similar height, similar clothes and similar features in general. They differed however, in one respect. One drawing was of a healthy child with no disfigurement or obvious impediment. Another depicted an obese child. The remaining four depicted children with some level of physical impairment. One was in a wheelchair with a blanket covering both legs. Another was holding crutches with a brace on their left leg. One had their left hand missing and finally, one had a facial disfigurement on the left side of their face. Boys were shown pictures of boys, and girls were shown pictures of girls. The teachers showed the pupils all six pictures and asked them to circle the picture of the person they liked most. That picture was then removed and the process repeated until all pictures were rated. The researchers then assigned a value to each picture for each child where one was the most liked drawing and six was the least liked drawing. Both boys and girls rated the healthy child the best (average 2.0). They ranked the four drawings of children with apparent physical abnormalities more or less the same (from 3.4 to 3.6). Boys tended to dislike functional disabilities while girls tended to least like appearance-related disabilities. However, the drawing of the obese child ranked worst with a mean score of 5.2 and this was the case for both boys and girls. The rankings were more or less the same in 1961 as they were in 2003. This very clear bias against the obese in children as young as ten to twelve emanates from parents, schools, the media, and just about every facet of society. The subject has been reviewed in depth by academics from Yale and they begin with an analysis of the data on obesity in employment settings.

All studies available on the topic show that obese persons are less likely to be hired compared to normal weight job applicants. Many techniques have been used to gauge attitudes to prospective employees from fictional CVs where weight is given to videotapes with the same actors manipulated to look either slimmer or fatter. In all instances, the fatter the applicant the less likely they were to be judged fit for the job in question.[3] They were deemed to lack self-discipline, to have low supervisory potential, poor personal hygiene, poor professional appearance and to be less neat, less productive, less ambitious, less disciplined and less determined. Obese applicants were judged to be more suited to jobs that did not involve face-to-face contact with clients. Even when obese persons are hired, they fare worse in terms of remuneration and promotion. For example, the US National Longitudinal Survey shows that obese women earned 12% less than non-obese women. Obese men don't merit such economic discrimination but they are more likely to work in non-professional jobs and are less likely to hold senior management positions. Bias against the obese in promotion is also well documented. In one study, managers were asked to rate the suitability of hypothetical candidates for promotion with certain disabilities or health problems: obesity, poor vision, depression, colon cancer, diabetes, arm amputation, facial burns or no disability. Guess who lost out most? The obese applicant, of course![4] The final act of prejudice against the obese is of course dismissal and many instances have been documented. One study of severely obese subjects showed that 17% reported being dismissed because of their weight. This has led on occasions to court proceedings and in most cases the judicial system has found bias against the obese as a basis for dismissal. For example, Agency Rent-a-Car Systems, Inc. dismissed Joseph Gimello despite Mr Gimello having an exemplary employment record.[5] In many instances where a dismissal is directly related to obesity, it is down to some arbitrary cut-off point in body weight, above which adequate work performance is deemed to be unattainable. One area where the courts have accepted a high body weight as an impediment to meeting employment duties is in the airline business. Understandably, there is often a maximum height restriction and weight is generally required to be proportionate to height and not impede the ability of a cabin crew member to wear the standard safety harness.

The next areas considered in the Yale-based review were medical and health settings and they concluded that health professionals share general cultural anti-fat attitudes. In one study, physicians were asked to identify patient characteristics that aroused certain feelings of discomfort, reluctance or dislike.[6] Drug addiction, alcoholism and mental illness ranked in the top three with obesity fourth. Doctors simply cannot hack obesity. The many studies of the attitude of physicians to the obese elicit the following descriptive adjectives: poor hygiene, noncompliance, dishonesty, poor self-control, lazy, lacking will power and so on. Almost 90% believed that obesity was a form of compensation due to lack of love or attention and 70% attributed obesity to emotional problems. Nurses didn't fare to well either. One third of nurses in one study would prefer not to care for an obese person and, in another, a quarter agreed or agreed strongly that caring for an obese patient repulsed them. That same sample revealed that one in eight nurses would prefer not to touch an obese person. Not exactly a Florence Nightingale model.[7]

One might imagine that dietitians and nutritionists would fare best when it came to bias against obesity. Regrettably that wasn't what was found. One study used a well-established tool to measure this issue. The 'Fat Phobia Scale' uses 14 pairs of opposing adjectives to describe obesity such as lazy/industrious, fast/slow or attractive/unattractive. The scoring system is such that if all the adjectives used to describe obese people were negative, a value of five would be assigned. In the event that obesity was associated with all favourable versions of the adjectives, the score would be one. The dietitians and nutritionists scored 3.8. This is higher than the average for a large sample of the general population (3.6) and if a value of 1.4 is used to classify people as having a low level of fat phobia, then only 1.4% of nutritionists and dietitians fell in this category.[8]

All in all, this review casts a very poor light on the caring professions in relation to obesity. Attitudes are one thing but actions that arise from such attitudes are what really hurt the obese. To begin with, appointment cancellation is far more common among the obese.[9] One third of those with clinical obesity and half of those with morbid obesity delayed or cancelled appointments and one study showed that obese women are much less likely to seek cancer screening checks. Physicians report spending just under 30% less time with obese patients and many deem such consultations to be a waste of their time. In one study, medical students examined virtual patients who were short of breath. If this was associated with a virtually obese patient, then the advice was four times more likely to involve lifestyle changes and five times less likely to involve medications to manage the problem. Patient management can also send out a very negative message to the obese. Blood pressure cuffs and patient gowns intended for the normal weight are of little use to the obese so a fuss is made to go somewhere to find a larger cuff or gown and that reinforces the bad experience of the obese patient. Chairs in waiting rooms that have armrests also send out a negative message to the obese for whom such chairs are either unusable or uncomfortable. It is unthinkable that a family doctor's practice might not have proper wheelchair access for the physically impaired or not have Braille facilities for the visually impaired. No such consideration is given to the obese. Why would they? Doctors, their nurses and receptionists generally have a fat phobia and believe all the negative connotations about the obese, including those that lay the blame on the personal shortcomings of the obese patient.

Those who are overweight find seating a problem in cinemas, theatres, buses, trains and planes and many legal battles have ensued in this regard. In one famous case, Ms Pamela Hollowich was asked to buy a second seat to accommodate her larger size and was warned that an armed guard would escort her off the plane if she attempted to board the aircraft. Greyhound, the large bus company, asked an overweight lady to leave the bus because she took up two seats. When she refused to leave, she was arrested and charged with disorderly conduct, a charge that was subsequently dropped. Other legal cases have arisen in restaurant and in theatre settings where obese persons were not accommodated with suitable seats. As the Yale review points out, there seems to be no problem with wheelchair bound individuals or pregnant women in the case of transport seating.

Eating Disorder

In a world where body weight is dominated by obesity, eating disorders lurk in the long grass, utterly anonymous except for those affected by these conditions, directly or indirectly, or by those who treat those so afflicted. Fasting to induce severe thinness is nothing new and it was a very common occurrence among strictly religious females. Catherine of Siena is a very famous example of what was called anorexia mirabilis whereby women in religious orders would starve themselves to an emaciated state for reasons of piety. In later years the Catholic church deemed such women to be bewitched and they met the usual fate of such. Many physicians began to diagnose self-imposed thinness associated with nervous disease and in 1873 Sir William Gull, physician to Queen Victoria (and popularly believed to have been Jack the Ripper), published a paper on what he called anorexia nervosa. Today, anorexia nervosa is only one of several eating disorders now defined in the *Diagnostic and Statistical Manual of Mental Disorders*, Fifth Edition.

Eating disorders are not defined by some single measure such as BMI for obesity. They are very complex conditions and to do justice to this very sensitive topic I have opted to transcribe directly from the website of ANRED (Anorexia Nervosa and Related Eating Disorders) the definitions of the main eating disorders and some lesser known ones.[10] ANRED is a non-profit organisation that is dedicated to the provision of information on eating disorders through their award-winning website. Below are profiles of three fictional girls covering the three main eating disorders (anorexia, bulimia nervosa and binge eating disorder) followed by an outline of the newly accepted condition 'eating disorder not specified'. I end with an unofficial condition, which describes people with an obsession with health eating, orthorexia nervosa.

Anorexia Nervosa
Laura refuses to maintain a normal weight for her age and height. She is obsessed with her image and is convinced she is fat even though she is frightfully skin and bone. She is terrified of gaining weight. She should weigh eight stone (51 kilograms) for her height but actually weighs 6.5 stone (41 kilograms). She has stopped menstruating. Laura is depressed, socially isolated of her own choice and has an array of strange eating habits, assigning foods and meals into categories such as 'safe' and 'dangerous'. She shuns normal responsibility for her age and is highly dependent on her family.

Bulimia Nervosa
Sandra is a massive binger on food but feels out of control of herself when eating. She uses tricks such as vomiting, laxatives, exercise and fasting to dump the calories she has binged on. She diets even when she isn't binging and then

becomes very hungry leading to another cycle of binging. She loves being super thin. She occasionally shoplifts and abuses her credit card. She is very fond of alcohol and will use mind-altering drugs if available. You would not know she had a weight problem just looking at her and she is like a lot thin girls her age. However, she is lonely, depressed and ashamed. Because she feels unworthy, she will not easily talk about her feelings which will include anxiety, depression, self-doubt and deeply buried anger.

Binge Eating Disorder

Thelma eats frequently and repeatedly and like Sandra, feels out of control in so doing. She can either eat rapidly, secretly or she may nibble or snack all day. She has a history of dieting but failing at these diets and is guilty and ashamed of her binge eating. She is depressed but unlike Sandra, she does not regularly vomit to control her weight or abuse laxatives. Those with this eating disorder may have a family problem with weight and may diet in a drastic way and then binge. Thelma will frequently eat for emotional reasons, which she uses to avoid threatening situations and to numb emotional pain.

Eating Disorders Not Otherwise Specified (ED-NOS)

This is now an official diagnosis introduced into the psychiatric lexicon. The phrase describes atypical eating disorders, including situations in which a person meets all but a few of the criteria for a particular diagnosis. What the person is doing with regard to food and weight is neither normal nor healthy. It is not a formal diagnosis even though it is a formally recognised condition. The behaviours are usually a part of anorexia nervosa, bulimia, or obsessive-compulsive disorder. The person repeatedly exercises beyond the requirements for good health (anorexia athletica) and may be a fanatic about weight and diet. A person with ED-NOS may steal time to exercise from work, school and relationships, and will focus on the challenge, forgetting that physical activity can be fun. Self-worth is defined in terms of performance and is rarely or never satisfied with athletic achievements. Victory is not savoured but simply drives the sufferer on to the next challenge immediately. This excessive behaviour is justified by a distorted image of himself or herself as a 'special' elite athlete.

Orthorexia Nervosa

Unlike the preceding conditions, this is not an official eating disorder diagnosis, but the concept is useful. The name was coined by Steven Bratman who described a pathological fixation on eating 'proper' or 'pure' or 'superior' food. People with orthorexia nervosa feel superior to others who eat 'improper' food, which might include non-organic or junk foods and items found in regular grocery stores, as opposed to health food stores. Orthorexics obsess over what to eat, how much to eat, how to prepare food 'properly', and where to obtain 'pure' and 'proper' foods. Eating the 'right' food becomes an important, or even the primary, focus of life. One's worth or goodness is seen in terms of what one does or does not eat. Personal values, relationships, career goals and friendships become less important than the quality and timing of what is consumed.

Frequency of Eating Disorders

Trying to estimate the frequency of eating disorders is fraught with difficulty. Not only are the diagnostic criteria complex but these conditions are often very private and held in secret by those suffering them. Measuring clinical cases grossly underestimates the scale of the problem. Surveying the population for data on such conditions will be frustrated by a high degree of under-reporting. Nonetheless, attempts have to be made to gain some idea of the scale of the problem. For The National Eating Disorders Association in the US the following top-line statistics apply:

- The lifetime incidence of anorexia nervosa among women is 0.5 to 3.7%, that of bulimia nervosa is 1.1 to 4.2% and for other eating disorders combined (mainly binge eating) it is between 2 and 5%.
- Up to 30 million people in the US of all ages and genders suffer from an eating disorder.
- Among teenagers, 50% of girls and 30% of boys use inappropriate means of weight control such as skipping meals, fasting, smoking, vomiting, and use of diuretics and laxatives.
- Among college-aged women, about 30% of all dieters progress to adopt these inappropriate slimming habits.[11]

Eating disorders should never become a reason to stop combatting obesity since their most severe forms are ancient and pre-date the modern epidemic of obesity. But we do need to be conscious of eating disorders and we do need to spend time and money in both prevention and management. The stigmatisation of obesity is a different matter. It represents a total casting of guilt on the overweight and fat person and implies a great level of superiority among those of us who are not overweight. It is a widespread but shameful condition for it ignores the most important features I have repeatedly highlighted in this book, namely contentment and happiness. We who cast this disgraceful and judgemental stigma feel smug. But in the next chapter I set out to look at all the players in obesity and try to see just how holy they all are. Few, you will see, survive this appraisal.

CHAPTER ELEVEN

Obesity: Politics, Players and Ploys

All of the great controversies and concerns of mankind are pushed this way and that way by diverse advocates and their followers. Obesity is no different. There are distinguished professors who speak in dire tones about obesity and its cost to human health. There are others, such as myself, who are a little sceptical about some aspects of the problem. There are journalists who have made food, health and obesity their specialty and yet again, there are journalists who differ in how they see the causes, the consequences and the cures of obesity. There are non-governmental organisations reflecting every viewpoint. There is a very vocal and defensive food industry and a very influential World Health Organization. In this chapter, I want to put all of these advocacy groups under the microscope and to parse out their driving forces. Before doing so, it would be worthwhile to consider how individuals acquire particular points of view and how and why those with similar points of view align themselves into groups of common interest that set out to promulgate their collective view of the world and to go head-to-head with those who see the world differently.

To this end, I rely heavily on Jonathan Haidt's acclaimed book: *The Righteous Mind: Why Good People Are Divided by Politics and Religion*.[1] Haidt concurs with Daniel Kahneman's System 1 and 2 of decision-making that I have referred to many times throughout this book.[2] Haidt's first message is: 'Intuition comes first, strategic reasoning second.' In effect he is saying that the positions that people take on political and moral issues are not normally the result of exhaustive research and soul searching. They are simply intuitive. All of the mental gymnastics and soul searching that then ensues is not to challenge the initial intuitive decision but to justify it. So where does this intuitive thinking come from? Nobody would argue that it is a random choice and the popular view would be that the home environment makes it very likely but not certain that individuals will adopt the world views of their parents. However, a growing body of thought would now argue that genetics play a significant role in shaping how people see the world. Using twin studies where identical twins share identical genomes and where non-identical twins share no more genetic material than non-twin siblings, it is possible, as was pointed out in chapter six, to separate out the role of genetics as opposed to the role of a shared (the home, similar schools or sports clubs) and unshared environment (different leisure interests and thus different clubs and groups) in shaping attitudes. When asked for their views on 28 attitudes and beliefs, there was a far higher concordance among identical twins than among non-identical twins.[3] However, when the inherited factor was compared to the shared and unshared environment the average percentage of variation was as follows: 32% for the genetic factor, 16% for the shared environment, mainly the home, and 53% for the unshared environment. Thus Haidt points out that genes lead people in certain directions. If your genes result in you embracing novelty, variety and diversity and to be less sensitive to signs of threats, then you are more likely, but by no means certain, to become a liberal. That is the genetic dimension. The second major point Haidt makes is that we are 'groupish'. We are 90% chimpanzee (cooperative) and 10% bee (selfish). We have evolved to work in groups for a common purpose. So if you have inherited a liberal draft brain then you are quite likely to go on to embrace a liberal political party or comparable organisation where that liberalism becomes powerfully reinforced. As Haidt puts it: 'Once people join a political team, they get ensnared in its moral matrix. They see confirmation of their grand narrative everywhere, and it's difficult – perhaps impossible – to convince them that they are wrong if you argue with them outside the moral matrix.' The same is true of groups who espouse some world view on the causes, consequences and cures of obesity. I grew up with very liberal parents so my brain was soft-wired toward liberal viewpoints and as I moved in my career, I was most unlikely to align myself with those who had a less liberal view of public health nutrition and obesity. Others have a more conservative view around obesity. Understanding how we develop our world views and how, through advocacy groups, we foster common world views simply helps us understand that all of those engaged in the debate on how obesity was caused and how it will be solved, are acting out of their own sense of moral and political values. Such an understanding helps us see the human side of this debate. Maybe, a greater understanding of such values among competing groups might help improve dialogue and might reduce the level of entrenchment on all sides. So, now let us consider the different groups involved and probe into their behaviour beginning with scientists.

Scientists and their Journals

Roger Pielke in his book *The Honest Broker: Making Sense of Science in Policy and Politics* classifies scientists into four groups.[4] The first is the 'Pure Scientist' who is wired to his or her laboratory and who has no interest in getting involved with time-wasting policy issues. The second is the 'Science Arbiter'. Such scientists will leave the lab to help tackle policy issues but do so in a low-key way, always avoiding the public limelight. The third group is classified as the 'Honest Broker of Policy Alternatives' and this group engages fully in the regulatory process but does so with a minimum of world view baggage. Scientists in this group let the data inform their collective opinion. The fourth group is entitled 'The Issue Advocate' and this group is agenda laden. They actively seek out involvement in regulatory matters and frequently are the ones who promote the establishment of some expert committee to act within one of the governmental or international agencies. They are likely to have a say in the selection of experts to sit on the advisory committee and they are darlings of the media and are often very well connected to key politicians. They also have a very big impact on funding agencies and on the developing views of younger scientists. They are very powerful. So when we look at scientists, we can see human 'groupish' tendencies as Haidt predicts and this emergence of views across the spectrum of obesity causes and consequences gives rise to factions who compete to shape policy. However, 'The Issue Advocates' have, as one would expect, the biggest say in the debate.

Jonathan Haidt also pointed out that within groups, we still retain selfishness – 90% chimpanzee and 10% bee. This selfishness drives the need to 'publish or perish' for scientific capital is measured in scientific output in the form of peer-reviewed papers and the extent to which these papers are cited by other authors. In the relentless pursuit of publications, scientists can often be just a little bit less than honest. Researchers at the University of Alabama in the US have looked at how scientists report other researchers' data. They took two published papers on obesity.[5] In the first example, the authors looked at an intervention study to decrease sugar-sweetened beverages in adolescents and concluded that after 12 months of intervention, there was no significant change in Body Mass Index. However, there was a significant difference in the percentage of overweight and obese subjects between the intervention group and the control group. In other scientific papers 165 authors cited the resultant paper. Of these, only 13% accurately reported the findings of this intervention study. 64% were mildly misleading in the way they presented the original findings of the intervention study. In effect, this 64% of citing authors mention the differences between groups in percentage overweight and obese but failed to mention the fact that there was no change between the groups in average BMI. 18% were explicitly misleading in the way they cited the data of the original intervention study. They described the effect of BMI as being significant when in fact it wasn't. The second case study was also an intervention study in adolescents looking again at how a reduction in sugar-sweetened beverages would influence body weight over six months compared to a control group. The authors again found no effect on average BMI between the two groups. They then selected a sub-group with a high initial BMI and noted an effect. Some 41 scientists cited this second case in their own papers. 33% accurately reported the findings. 30% were classified as 'patently misleading' because they stated that the effect of the intervention was significant on mean BMI without ever referring to the fact that this was not actually significant in the original paper. In effect they mentally noted the effect in a small sub-group with the higher BMI and then mentally and wrongly transferred that to mean BMI. 37% who cited the paper were classified as 'mildly misleading over-positive' by emphasising the small sub-group effect and ignoring the non-significant effect in the total sample. This group, led by Professor David Allison, also looked at other areas of honesty in scientific reporting. As previously pointed out, the only studies that can truly claim to show cause and effect are those in which a proposed cause of some obesity-related factor is altered over a period of time (intervention group), while another group is treated identically but without the primary intervention (control group).

Most of the studies linking diet, lifestyle and obesity involve observational studies. Thus at a given time point, a population is studied and factors which differ between the overweight and obese are identified. For example, a study might examine a large database to see if sleep duration differs between the obese and the lean. If it does, the most the authors can say is that there appears to be some link between, let us say, shortest length of sleep and obesity. They simply cannot infer from such observational studies that short-ness of sleep duration causes obesity. But do they? Allison's group looked at the four leading journals (*Obesity, The American Journal of Clinical Nutrition, The International Journal of Obesity* and *The Journal of Nutrition*) that publish papers on diet, lifestyle and obesity. They examined all articles published in 2006 amounting to 1,617 of which 525 were observational studies.[6] Of these, 31% used causal language in the title or abstract and, in nine times out of ten, journalists read only the abstract. It didn't matter whether the research was funded by industry or governmental agencies. The average misuse of causal language in observational studies was the same. These two examples of stretching the data in papers they cite and inappropriately inferring causality from observational studies raise serious concerns for editors of scientific journals. It also raises concerns about the transmission of data from researchers to the mass media – where the public gets most of their information. It is to the mass media that we now turn.

Hardly a day goes by without some part of the mass media reporting on some new finding in the field of food, diet and health. Typically, it is announced that 'Professor Ivan Ego' of the 'University of Numbers' has published a major new study in the *'International Journal of Cancer Fiction'* that shows a direct link between the consumption of pulled pork and the incidence of cancer of the eyelashes. The journalist concerned didn't come across this paper after an exhaustive trawl of the scientific literature. No, the journalist faithfully reproduced the contents of a press release issued by either the 'University of Numbers' or maybe the *'International Journal of Cancer Fiction'*. Universities and scientific and medical journals vie for headlines that make their presidents and editors feel good and which enhance their reputation in a highly competitive world. Professor David Allison of the University of Alabama, in a centre funded by the National Institute of Health, has published data which look at the spin that can be put on research findings by universities, hospitals and medical journals. Here are three examples from his study.[7]

Case 1

This was a study which lasted two years and involved 224 overweight or obese adolescents, half of whom were given supplies of bottled water or diet beverages plus support telephone calls every two weeks for the first year of the study (intervention group). The authors wrote that the primary outcome of the study, as outlined in advance of the commencement of the study on the US clinical trials website, was the change in weight at two years. There was no statistically significant difference between the control group and the intervention group in this primary outcome of body weight. There was a difference in BMI between the two groups at the end of year one but that was not the *a priori* primary outcome. The Children's Hospital at the University of Harvard in Boston, where the study was coordinated issued a press release which stated:

Children's intake of sugar-sweetened drinks – sodas, sports drinks, 'juice drinks', iced teas, lemonades and punches – has surged in recent decades, in step with the rise in childhood obesity. Now, in the March issue of *Pediatrics*, researchers from Children's Hospital Boston report that a novel intervention to limit consumption of sugary drinks – home deliveries of noncaloric beverages – had a beneficial effect on weight loss.

Case 2

In this school-based study lasting 12 months, an intervention group of adolescents received intensive counselling to reduce their intake of sugary drinks in three sessions, with the use of educational aids of various sorts including a sample of a tooth in a fizzy drink to convey the dangers of such! The authors wrote that after 12 months there was no significant change in the differences in BMI between the control and intervention group. In fact, the study failed to reduce (at a statistically significant level) the intakes of carbonated drinks, with or without added sugar. The *British Medical Journal*, which published the study, issued a press release stating: 'Fewer fizzy drinks can prevent childhood obesity . . . discouraging children from consuming fizzy drinks can prevent excessive weight gain according to new research available at BMJ.com.'

Case 3

In a third study, 318 overweight and obese subjects were divided into three groups. Two of these were given either bottled water or diet beverages and participated in monthly weigh-in sessions and group counselling. The intervention group was treated identically except that they were not given free bottled water or diet beverages. Weight loss occurred in all three groups and there was no statistically significant difference between these groups. The University of North Carolina's press release states: 'Making a simple substitution of water or diet soft drinks for drinks with calories can help people lose 4 to 5 pounds, a new study at the University of North Carolina at Chapel Hill shows.'

It would be wrong to say that the press releases absolutely ignored the main findings. Naturally, the relevant press officer sifted through an abstract or conclusions and opted for the juicy bits of the study. That is their job and it is to be expected that journalists will take these press releases and make a good story from it. The average citizen reads it and their views, for or against, are confirmed. The guilty parties are the scientists who completed the study and who did not correct the press release. Quite simply, this sort of publicity is good for the university or scientific journal involved and this is a very competitive field. So, what's wrong with a little exaggeration of the truth? The problem is that when junk data are reiterated time after time, junk data become true data and to question them, is verging on scientific heresy. When junk data get to this level, it is inevitably incorporated into popular, best-selling but nonetheless junk books delivering dire warnings about this food or that food sector in obesity and the cycle continues. All this exposure and all the attendant citizens' concerns about diet and health, together with the help of 'The Issue Advocate' scientist, drive political thinking and policy action. But the perceived global doyenne of truth in public health is the World Health Organization (WHO), the next group for examination.

The World Health Organization

In 2007, a paper was published in the medical journal the *Lancet* that sought to study how the WHO expert panels reach their conclusions, which are profoundly important in shaping global policy on public health.[8] The study, conducted jointly between the Norwegian Centre for Health Services and the Centre for Health Economics at McMaster University in Canada, and funded by the EU, concluded that systematic reviews were rarely used and the favoured way of developing a report was to use an expert committee or individual experts. One interview among the 29 directors or equivalents commented thus: 'There is a tendency to get people around a table and get consensus – everything they do has a scientific part and a political part. This usually means you go to the lowest common denominator or the views of a "strong" person at the table.' This criticism was bad enough but worse was to come. Two papers were published subsequently in the *Lancet*, one by researchers looking at insecticide treated anti-malarial bed nets and another looking at child mortality. For the first paper, the authors outline the success of the programme but, importantly, they also outline some important uncertainties in the data. The WHO received drafts of the data and ahead of the *Lancet* publication, issued a press release claiming that the data 'ends the debate about how to deliver long-lasting insecticidal nets'. The second paper from researchers at Harvard and Queensland universities reported disappointing progress in the rate of reduction of childhood mortality. UNICEF contacted the *Lancet* about the paper but after considerable consultation with individual experts the *Lancet* decided to publish and informed UNICEF of the intended data of the publication. UNICEF then fast tracked the publication of its annual *State of the World's Children Report* and made claims contrary to the paper. These two actions by the UN agencies caused the *Lancet* to pen an editorial which concluded thus:

> But the danger is that by appearing to manipulate science, breach trust, resist competition and reject accountability, WHO and UNICEF are acting contrary to scientific norms that one would have expected UN technical agencies to uphold. Worse, they risk inadvertently corroding their own long-term credibility.[9]

Scornful criticism for a top class medical journal!

The UN moves slowly and thus in 2012, in response to such scathing criticism, it issued a specific handbook for guideline development and established a Guideline Review Committee to be involved in evaluating all subsequent guidelines. Central to this process was the internationally accepted approach to the development of guidelines called the GRADE (Grading of Recommendations Assessment, Development and Evaluation) process. GRADE is used to evaluate confidence in the effect of some action or intervention and classifies this confidence as high, moderate, low or very low. If there is more than one effect possible, the overall grading is based on the weakest measure of confidence. In addition to the strength of evidence on outcomes from actions or interventions, GRADE also rates the overall recommendations as strong or conditional. An international panel set out to examine how guidelines and recommendations of the WHO adhered to the GRADE system since its introduction in 2007 up to the year 2012.[10] A total of 167 recommendations were found and reviewers worked in pairs to evaluate adherence to GRADE guidelines. Of the guidelines deemed to be strong, 56% were found to have low or very low confidence in estimates. Only 17% had high confidence in estimates. Turning to the 167 recommendations that were considered weak, 85% were indeed based on low to very low confidence in the estimates of the effect of the action or intervention. Thus for example, 100% of the strong recommendations were found to be based on low to very low effects estimates for guidelines on nutrition and influenza. Half of the recommendations in the area of maternal and reproductive health, child health, HIV/AIDS and TB was deemed to be strong recommendations based on low to very low confidence in the outcome effects.

The same set of researchers went one step further in a follow up paper.[11] Sometimes, expert committees have to make judgements. The confidence in the true significance effect estimate might not be as strong as they'd like but the expert committee feels that a strong recommendation is warranted for whatever reason. These are called discordant recommendations and GRADE recognises five situations where a discordant recommendation is warranted. Given the very high number of strong recommendations with weak effect evidence observed in the previous study, the researchers set out to see how many of these met any one of the five situations, which GRADE allows a discordant recommendation. Only 16% of the discordant recommendations met any one of the five situations where GRADE accepts a discordant recommendation. In all, 84% of the discordant recommendations did not meet the GRADE guidelines. 46% of the discordant recommendations (strong recommendation but low supporting evidence) should have been classified as simply conditional recommendations. These two papers show that the WHO still has a long way to go to meet reasonable levels of scientific integrity. It may well be that expert panels make strong recommendations based on weak evidence of effect because otherwise their recommendations would be ignored. The problem is that in many countries, a strong recommendation from the WHO is the first step in the development of national policies and such is the respect that many national public health agencies have in the WHO and their guidelines that they go unquestioned. Anyone who has had dealings with large UN agencies knows that they are frequently short of resources and given that they answer to multiple national governments and to multiple non-governmental organisations, it is correct to have some level of understanding of their constraints. However, failure to rigorously embed their guidelines in the highest quality of science and the repeated issuing of strong recommendations based on weak to very weak evidence-based outcomes, means that they cannot be excused. They may keep most non-governmental activists happy but in the long term, global trust is more important. It is hard won and easily lost.

Non-Governmental Organisations

Who are these non-governmental activists (NGOs) and what is their role in civil society? For these purposes, it is easier to consider NGOs as a whole and not simply NGOs with an obesity agenda. To do so, I draw heavily on a paper by Dr Paul Jepson at the Oxford University Centre for the Environment.[12] He argues that three critical points determined the rise of global NGOs since the early 1990s. Firstly, there was a perceived need to create an international civil society that could work with and challenge the international agencies. To that point, such agencies answered to governmental organisations and not to civil society. Secondly, there was a move toward the rolling back of the state services, effectively ceding policy development to NGOs. A simple example was the huge growth in 'Heart Foundations' that effectively took on what governments should have taken on. Thirdly, there was the recognition that the everyday lives of ordinary citizens were now being determined by non-accountable trans global corporations, by the anonymous and poorly understood international 'markets' and by inaccessible inter-governmental organisations such as the World Trade Organisation. The advent of the NGOs was clearly a good thing for democracy, a good thing for civil society and a point of reassurance among ordinary citizens that now, there was a consumer-friendly, powerful force acting as a counterbalance to the anonymous forces of capitalism. Now in putting NGOs under the microscope in this chapter, the reader must understand their scale. Taking environmental NGOs (ENGOs), their economic scale is enormous. The largest ENGO is The Nature Conservancy which has assets in the region of $6.5 billion.[13] The World Wildlife Fund has assets in the region of $120 million,[14] and the Royal Society for the Protection of Birds in the UK had a net income of just £100 million in 2014.[15] This is not a criticism: it is merely to assert that the large NGOs are huge. By and large, their income is comprised of individual member subscriptions, philanthropic donations, private sector gifts and public sector grants.

When it comes to accountability, that phrase is usually confined to financial and governance credibility. For example, *The Washington Post* in 2003 published a series of articles on The Nature Conservancy revealing land assets of €2.73 billion.[16] That year we saw the Enron collapse and so The Nature Conservancy finances and governance came under intense scrutiny leading to major reforms of its structures, an action that seriously shook the NGO world.[17] Reform of NGO accountability and governance might simply involve importing such norms from the corporate world but as Jepson points out, such norms may not be suitable for global NGOs. However global NGOs manage their financial and governmental accountability, there remains the issue of scientific integrity and to date, there has been no systematic review of how NGOs, including industry-funded NGOs, manage their scientific evaluations according to best international practice. NGOs are a fine example of human 'groupiness' as outlined by Jonathan Haidt where persons of like minds gather to bolster, defend and promulgate their point of view. They are here to stay and we are better for their presence. Governance and financial accountability need to be addressed and, ultimately, all those issuing scientific opinions, whether the WHO, obesity-linked NGOs or industry-funded NGOs, need to adhere to the highest standard of scientific rigour.

Industry

The food industry is the final group to be placed under the microscope in this chapter. US Oxfam has in fact done this, as they see it, in the programme 'Behind the Brands'.[18] The scoring system is thus: good (8–10), fair (6–7), some progress (4–5), poor (2–3) and very poor (0–1). All of this is corporate-directed and tells us nothing about the contribution of these top ten food companies to nutrition. However, the implication from the table below and many other NGO reports on the food industry is that the focus of the global food problem of obesity lies firmly in the hands of these multinationals. I am afraid that I am going to dispute this and thus shift the scale of the problem from an easy issue of just ten culpable candidates to hundreds of thousands of possible offenders.

Company	Land	Women	Farmers	Workers	Climate	Transpar-ency	Water	Score %
Unilever	7	5	8	8	9	7	6	71
Nestlé	8	5	7	6	8	7	7	69
Coca-Cola	8	6	2	6	6	5	5	54
Pepsico	7	2	2	3	6	5	5	43
Mars	2	5	4	4	6	4	3	40
Mondeéz (formerly Kraft Foods)	3	6	4	3	4	4	2	37
Kellogg's	2	3	2	2	7	5	3	34
Danone	2	1	2	3	6	5	3	31
General Mills	2	2	2	2	5	4	5	31
Associated British Foods	3	2	3	4	4	3	2	30

Let me start with other industries. First the mobile or cell phone market Samsung, Nokia, Apple, LG, ZTE and Huawei, together account for almost 60% of global sales, globally dominating the phone business. The same is true of other markets: aircraft (Boeing, Airbus), cars (Ford, Volkswagen, Mercedes, Toyota, Nissan, General Motors, Peugeot, Hyundai, Kia etc.), televisions (Samsung, LG, Sony, Panasonic, Sharp, Vizio, Philips, Toshiba, Mitsubishi etc.) and hotels (Radisson, Best Western, Hilton, Sheraton, Westin, Mercure,

Novotel, Ramada, Marriot, Crown Plaza etc). Now let me take the last group and ask a simple question. Of all the hotels in Ireland, how many belong to this international group? According to my calculations about 10% belong to this international set of hotels, the rest (say 80% to be conservative) being local hotels. The same is exactly true of foods and therein lies the challenge. If I just take one everyday product, mayonnaise, I find that the database Euro Pages lists all of 43 companies in the EU which manufacture mayonnaise and this excludes the big ones such as Hellman's.[19]

Now, using wider EU data, let me show you the true landscape of the manufacturing food sector. The total turnover of the EU food manufacturing sector is €1 trillion. It accounts for 16% of all EU manufacturing and it employs 4.1 million people. So the EU food sector is huge. But now consider the players. Some 99% are small to medium enterprises which means that they employ less than 250 persons and have a turnover less than €50 million. They account for half of the EU food manufacturing turnover and they employ two thirds of all persons employed in that sector. The vast majority you have never heard of, since food SMEs generally operate within very limited geographic regions typically serving one province and several cities. In general, those who innovate in food tend to do so in a very local up to national market. A tiny fraction hit the global market. So, 1% of the food manufacturing industry in the EU is comprised of large companies who might feature on some top 100 list but they account for only half the turnover and a third of the employment in this sector. The very large multinationals are actively engaged in very high profile activities to enhance their image among an increasingly ethical financial investment sector. They have policies of reformulation to improve the nutritional quality of their products. They constantly pursue improved food chain sustainability, fair trade, the rights of women and children, water conservation, climate change factors and so on. And they are the brands that make most noise in television advertising and they are also the global face of the food sector. However, if the food chain is to be reformed to meet improved nutritional needs, it may help to highlight issues by activities such as Oxfam's 'Behind the Brand' campaign and it may make food NGOs happy. But the reality is that they never heard of the 99% of the sector that are the minnows that dominate the food manufacturing sector. Their role in improving nutrition requires an entirely different strategy and, frankly, I don't see a lot of activity in this sphere. We will return to the food sector in the last chapter.

These are the main players in the food and health issues that dominate global and national debate on the obesity challenge to public health. To at least understand them might be the basis for dialogue and common strategies to address the problem of obesity. There is one further player, governments, and I will discuss their role in the final chapter of this book.

CHAPTER TWELVE

Weight Management: The Personal Perspective

From an evolutionary point of view, it made sense for people to be able to lose weight when times were hard and to return to normal weight when the food supply began to improve. Equally, it made sense in anticipation of seasonal food shortages ahead, that people could put on weight to survive the hard times, ultimately to return to the normal weight when conditions changed. This highly adaptive process enabled people to have the survival mechanisms to deal with all forms of adverse dietary conditions. The key point here is that there was a normal weight to which people returned following the loss or the gain of weight, and again, it made evolutionary sense to have this established weight that some-how, unbeknown to us, our bodies always defended. Throughout the history of man, nothing has changed in this regard and prior to any consideration of the dieting process to deal with excess body weight, it is necessary to explore the biology of this phenomenon of the body's apparent defence of a given body weight. Let's first consider weight gain, which as I have earlier stated is a stealth process since for the vast majority of people they simply wake up one day a little unhappy with their weight and ultimately find themselves ensnared in the grip of overweight and obesity. It is not at all a conscious decision and is 100% System 1 thinking. However, there are instances where weight gain becomes a very conscious effort and requires System 2 thinking with detailed planning of the optimal strategy to weight gain together with the continuous monitoring of the success of this process. Sumo wrestlers apparently maintain diets of 10,000 calories a day to achieve their professional objectives of body weight.[1] The women of the Efik tribe in Calabar in the south east of Nigeria, enter a fattening room prior to marriage where the day is spent gorging on six large meals a day with three massages in between and with plenty of sleep.[2] The older women teach the brides-to-be about housework, cooking, childcare and the like and they emerge from the fattening room in traditional dress, soon to meet their husband-to-be. A third group of weight gainers are Hollywood actors.[3] Vincent D'Onofrio holds the record of a gain of 70 pounds for the movie *Full Metal Jacket*. Close behind is Robert De Niro who gained 60 pounds for the movie *Raging Bull* and Renee Zellweger holds the record for actresses when she gained 30 pounds for her role in *Bridget Jones's Diary*. When an individual gains weight for a shortish period, which would correspond in evolutionary terms to say a season, there is every chance that given a period of restrained eating, this weight would return to normal. The problem is that if the weight gain persists beyond some reasonable time, the body readjusts its energy balance switch upwardly and, here is the catch, permanently. In other words the biological mechanisms at play make the decision as it were, that this weight increase is the new norm and now this new norm will be defended. The Hollywood actors and actresses who gained weight hopefully managed to do so such that a new control level wasn't established. The sumo wrestler and the bride-to-be from the Efik tribe in Nigeria sincerely hope that the body is re-booted to expect and to defend a higher body weight. This is the reason why so many people regain weight. Basically, the silent biological regulatory mechanisms of body weight control win out over the conscious (System 2) efforts to lose weight. The trouble for those for whom excess weight was unconsciously gained is that for many if not most, their weight control set point is permanently shifted upwards.

A second aspect of body weight biology needs to be considered. Since the objective of dieting is to consume fewer calories than expended, it is worth considering the energy expenditure side of caloric balance. There are three main components to energy expenditure. One is physical activity which was dealt with in chapter eight. For most sedentary people, this amounts to a mere 15% of total energy expenditure. A second is the thermic effect of food. This is the cost of the digestion of foods: the absorption, distribution, transport and storage of the nutrients in a meal. Typically, the value assigned for the thermic effect of food is 10% of total energy expenditure. The remaining energy expenditure is resting metabolism, which accounts for a staggering 75% of total caloric intake. Resting metabolic energy expenditure provides energy for vital organ function whether awake or asleep. It provides the energy needed for the pumping of the heart, the heaving of our lungs and the functioning of the brain, muscle, gut, spleen, pancreas, skeleton, thymus, kidneys and so on. Some people mistakenly believe that if an organ such as the gut is not doing its digestive and absorptive thing, then it requires no energy. That is not so. Every organ in the body is constantly being broken down and rebuilt, minute in minute out, hour in hour out, day in day out. So all our organs at all times require energy input and the totality of this demand is resting (or basal) metabolic rate.

In trying to understand some of the constraints that apply to dieting, it is necessary to consider two important aspects of resting metabolic rate. Knowledge of a person's weight and age can be used in equations developed by Professor Jeya Henry at the University of Singapore to estimate resting metabolic rate.[4] I weigh 110 kilograms and am aged 68 years at the time of writing. Thus these equations tell me that my resting metabolic rate is 1,875 calories per day. If I was sedentary, which I'm not, and these 1,875 calories from resting metabolic rate represents just 75% of my caloric expenditure, then my total daily energy expenditure would be 2,500 calories. So, if I opt to consume 1,500 calories a day on my diet, I'll have a daily energy deficiency of about 1,000 calories. Well it's not as easy as that. Because I've gone on a diet, the body quickly recognises a state of energy deficiency and so it does its evolutionary survival thing and it drops total daily resting metabolic rate. Effectively it 'turns down the revs' on the body's energy output and this happens very soon into dieting and will amount to about a 15% reduction in basal metabolic rate. Thus my resting metabolic rate now falls to 1,594 kilocalories giving me a new daily requirement of 2,125 calories. Thus if I want to retain a deficit of 1,000 calories, my daily caloric limit falls to just 1,125 calories. The adaptive fall in resting metabolic rate thus makes it more difficult to lose weight which is exactly what the fall is intended to do, an evolutionary adaptation against hard times.

There is a second area where we need to consider resting metabolic rate. Compare two men in their 40s one weighing 85 kilograms and the other weighing 125 kilograms. The former will need a daily caloric supply of 2,109 calories while the latter will need 2,733 calories. The difference is equivalent to a McDonald's burger and small French fries or its equal to a serving of a restaurant portion of spaghetti with a meat sauce such a bolognese. Thus when you next see a fat person eat more than average, bear in mind that their large body weight expends a greater amount of energy and that has to be balanced with a greater energy intake. The temptation as we have seen is to turn this higher caloric choice by a fat person into a judgement. Please don't. Be understanding. An appreciation of metabolic rate is central to understanding the challenges to weight management, which is where we now turn to.

I had a PhD student once, who was tall and slim. However, he had not always been so. As an undergraduate, he suffered the usual negative bias that is associated with overweight. He went on a diet and as he lost weight, he placed a

2-kilogram redbrick into a suitcase. As he got lighter, the suitcase got heavier and he only had to lift it to realise how important it was to keep that weight off. In his travels from undergraduate to postgraduate to employment, he took this case with him. Losing weight is easy. Keeping it off is very hard. In fact, the American Medical Association's Council on Scientific Affairs wrote: 'The 5 year cure rate for obesity is less than the 5 year cure rate for the worst cancer.'[5] So, you want to lose weight? Well the first thing you need to do is to sit down and think it through. A first question would be to ask if you had any of the adverse medical effects of overweight and obesity. Go to your doctor and get your blood pressure, blood cholesterol, blood glucose, blood uric acid and your liver function measured. If all of these come back fully normal, then unless you pursue matters further and have tests such as ECG or MRI scanning, then you have no urgent medical need to lose weight. If on the other hand you have some adverse effects of obesity, such as elevated blood pressure and blood cholesterol, then you now face a choice. You could forget about diet and seek a pharmacological solution to your health problems. The drugs will work, for sure. The question you have to ask yourself is: 'Will dieting work for me?' Dieting here doesn't mean a temporary weight loss; it means a lifetime weight loss. You have to recognise the fact that 50% of people who lose weight will have regained it in full within two years. So maintaining weight loss is no stroll in the park.

If you do decide to lose weight, you must first build in expectations of setbacks leading to small or somewhat larger weight regain. My strong advice is to get help from either a qualified specialist in weight management or organisations such as Unislim, Jenny Craig or Weight Watchers. You can of course buy yourself a copy of the latest 'branded diet' such as the Atkins Diet, the South Beach Diet, the Zone Diet or the Ornish Diet. Take your pick from the wonderful book by Louise Foxcroft, *Calories and Corsets*.[6] Recent research shows that these diets, which vary in their favourite calorie to shed (low fat or low carb) show no difference whatsoever in their weight loss performance.[7] A major multi-centre collaborative research product named 'POUNDLOST' compared four diets: low fat, high carbohydrate; low fat, high protein; high fat, low carbohydrate; high fat, high protein. In all, 811 overweight and obese persons took part. On average, the participants showed a 13-pound weight loss at six months and at two years had maintained an average of nine-pound weight loss. They lost one to three inches from their waist and there were no differences across dietary groups in feelings of fullness, craving or hunger nor were there differences in diet satisfaction. All in all, the extensive literature shows that caloric deficits are at the heart of successful weight loss.[8]

Before proceeding on my advice to those who want to lose weight, I'd like to give some words of warning: don't go to the health food shop and purchase pills for your weight loss. The regulation of body weight is such a complex biological system involving your brain, gut, muscles, liver, pancreas and so forth with an endless number of pathways involved. As a consequence the drug industry has struggled to come up with a drug that works consistently and safely. If the drug industry, so heavily regulated by regulatory watchdogs such as the US Food and Drugs Administration or the European Medicine Agency finds it hard to achieve a successful drug, you can be sure that all of the over-the-counter food supplements for weight loss lack any level of scientific rigour. Take for example the popular weight loss product CLA (conjugated linoleic acid). In studies with rats and mice, CLA appears to increase muscle mass and reduce fat mass. However, an expert opinion of the European Food Safety Authority concludes, as do all properly conducted reviews, that there is no evidence for such an effect in humans.[9] That doesn't stop the health food industry and some pharmacies from making claims as to the potential of CLA to reduce weight in humans. One simple illustration of the dangers of weight loss supplements, especially those purchased over the internet, was the inclusion of trace amounts of a banned weight loss drug. The drug's active ingredient was sibutramine and was previously marketed as Meridia. The drug was banned in 2010 because of adverse effects on the cardiovascular system. Unless prescribed by a medical doctor or a dietitian with prescriptive authority, don't buy weight loss pills. You will waste your money and potentially risk your health. Face up to reality. As Dolly Parton once said to the BBC talk show host Michael Parkinson: 'Honey, if you want to lose weight, get your head out of the slop bucket.' The advice I will give you is to first read three books, one on our food environment, one on choosing preparing low energy dense dishes and the third on exercise, specifically counting steps. All are written by highly regarded US academics with global reputations for their research output.

Let's start with Professor Brian Wansink of the University of Cornell and his book: *Mindless Eating: Why We Eat More Than We Think*.[10] He talks of the 'mindless margin', that is, 100 calories above or below your ideal caloric intake. Above or below that margin we are either knowingly gaining weight or consciously restricting caloric intake. The mindless margin is, as the name implies, a zone that we may be in but not really be aware that's where we are. He has many illustrations in his book of mindless eating so I will illustrate the principle with three examples. In his research facility they have a nice restaurant called The Spice Box. A meal here at either of the two sittings will cost $25 and it is very much fine dining. The researchers purchased several boxes of a $2 Charles Shaw wine popularly known as 'two buck chuck'. For one part of this study, the labels were removed and replaced with a label indicating that it was a Californian wine. The diners were told on arrival that they were getting a complimentary glass of fictional new wine from California. For the second part of the study, the same trick and treat was applied except that the diners were told that the wine was a new wine from Dakota. Now Dakota doesn't have a climate to grow wine but California does. When the diners finished, the researchers checked the plates to quantify leftovers in caloric terms. They also timed the duration of the meal. Those given the Californian wine consumed 11% more calories and lingered on average ten minutes longer at the table. Remember, it was the same food and the same wine but those given the Dakota labelled wine had it in their heads that this was not going to be a great meal. They ate less. This was mindless eating. In case you thought that they didn't like the Dakotan wine, they did. Both groups polished off the free large glass of wine. But the Californian labelled wine had a halo effect on the overall dining experience.

A second example relates to the great American feast that surrounds their Super Bowl, the cup final of American football. Two groups of MBA students were treated to free soft drinks (beer was charged for), free chicken wings and a big television to watch the game on. They had access to as many chicken wings as they liked and they could go back as often as they wished for additional helpings of wings. When they were finished eating a chicken wing, they put the bones in a bowl on the table. One group had their bowls replaced by a new clean bowl at four intervals throughout the night. The full bowl was returned to the kitchen to quantify the number of chicken wings eaten. For the other half, the bowls were not replaced and the bones simply accumulated. Those that had the bowls of bones removed ate 28% more than those who were left with the visual cue of a bowl full of bones.

The last example of mindless eating again involves students given free Chex Mix snacks. This time the subjects were graduate students who had taken part in a 90-minute class on how servings selected can be biased by the size of the container from which the food is taken. Once again, the study was done on a Super Bowl night and the rationale for this was to facilitate mindless eating where the focus is on the game. In one room the Chex Mix snacks were taken from two huge two-gallon containers. In another, they took their snacks from four half-gallon containers. When they got to the end of the line they were asked to fill in a questionnaire on Super Bowl commercials. They had only one place to put their bowl of snacks as they filled in the questionnaire and that was at a corner of the table. They didn't know that there was a sensitive weighing scale there to find out the serving weight of snacks they had chosen. Those who were offered snacks from the two-gallon containers chose 53% more than those who selected from the half-gallon containers. These students were not ignorant of the bias that originates from the size of the container from which food is selected. Nonetheless, they were guilty of mindless eating.

Once we accept that we tend to eat mindlessly, we can begin to do something about it. First, since we know that most people at most meals clean their plate, Professor Wansink advises that we put 20% less on our plate of all foods except vegetables where we should put 20% more on. He has established that this 20% will not be noticed. It won't make you hungrier in the normal course of events. It might not apply when we eat after a round of golf or a half marathon but in everyday life, that 20% isn't noticed. He also makes the point that in Japanese culture they select a quantity of food such that when it is eaten, they will no longer be hungry. In the US he points out that the intention is to select enough food to feel full at the end of the meal. He also argues that since we eyeball our intended quantity of food, we should put on the plate exactly what we intend to eat and not keep going back for seconds. In general, research shows that the one plate only approach will result in 14% less calories than repeatedly filling the plate.

Since mindless eating is mindless, anything that causes us to think might also cause us to eat more mindfully. To study this, he gave secretaries a treat for Secretaries Week, namely nicely covered dishes with chocolates in them. Half the dishes was clear and the other half was white. Both had lids so the secretaries with the white dishes could not eyeball the chocolates. Each evening the chocolates were counted and those eaten were replaced and that went on for two weeks. Those given the chocolates in the clear dishes ate 71% more than those for whom the chocolates were not visible. Once again, the eyes have it. Next they gave all secretaries chocolates in clear dishes. For each secretary, the location of the dish rotated into three different positions: the corner of the desk, the left hand drawer of the desk or in a filing cabinet six feet from the desk. When the dish was available on the desk, nine chocolates (225 calories) were eaten. If the desk drawer had to be opened to access the dish, six chocolates were eaten and if the secretary had to walk to the filing cabinet to get chocolates, then only four were eaten. That amounts to 125 less calories between the desktop and the filing cabinet. So whilst the eyes have it, their mindless impact on food choice can be interrupted if something is introduced to make the mind work. The slightest inconvenience provides those critical seconds to change one's mind. This is further illustrated in yet another of his studies. Subjects were given a packet of Pringles to eat to their satisfaction. In one case, every seventh Pringle was coloured red. In another case, every fourteenth was coloured red. For the final group there were no red Pringles. Where every seventh one was red, the number eaten was ten. Where every fourteenth Pringle was red, 15 Pringles were eaten. With no colour, 23 were eaten. Anything, be it a six-foot trip to the filing cabinet or a colour cue to spike the mind will help combat mindless eating. So Brian Wansink advises us to build some level of inconvenience into food choice. If you are fond of chocolates, put them into a screw-top jar. If you can buy something in bulk that can be frozen then freeze them in smaller containers. As will be seen again later in this chapter, keeping a record is an extremely useful tool. Professor Wansink recommends that it is best to select three things to do to avoid mindless eating. Use a small plate might be one, slow down and start and end last is another, and only serve vegetables 'family style', where each person chooses their own servings. The most important thing you will get from this book is not a diet but an understanding of mindless eating and really practical tips to limit this scourge.

For my second book I move to an actual diet book written by Professor Barbara Rolls from Pennsylvania State University.[11] She is a world authority on energy density, that is, the number of calories per gram of food. At the top end are oils and fats with nine calories per gram. At the other end is water with no calories per gram. So a dish that is high in fat (fried eggs, sausage and bacon) has a high energy density while a dish with a high water content (soup) has a low energy density. Professor Rolls's group studies energy density by painstakingly designing dishes that look the same, taste the same and smell the same but vary in the amount of energy on the plate. In order to study the feeling of satiety, she first gives her subjects a dish which will vary each day only in energy density (the pre-load dish) and then some time later, usually a few hours, the subjects are given access to a food (test meal) and are asked to eat until they are full. The following is a simple example.[12] On one occasion the subjects are given a casserole dish as the pre-load and then are given free access to the test meal. The next intervention uses the identical serving of the same casserole but this time the subjects drank 356 grams of water throughout the pre-load meal. The third arm of the study took the same amount of the same casserole and the same amount of water and blended them together into a soup. Compared to the day when the subjects ate the control (casserole only) pre-load, they consumed 100 calories less of the test meal when their pre-load was the soup.

Once again, we see how the visual dimension operates in determining how much food we eat. One could be critical of this and argue that the effect of energy density would wear off and that people would ultimately compensate for this. Well the Penn State researchers took that challenge into a pre-school setting in a two-day study.[13] Children aged three to five might not be as savvy as adults and therefore their food intake might be more determined by biology than by visual aspects. The researchers manipulated breakfast, lunch and afternoon snacks over a two-day period on two separate weeks. For one week the meals and snacks were high energy density (1.77 calories per gram) and on the other they were low energy density (1.32 calories per gram). They looked the same. To make sure that the researchers covered all foods eaten over the two days, they gave the children pre-packed dinner and snacks to take home but these did not vary in energy density. The total weight of food consumed over the two days was not influenced by energy intake (about 2,400 grams on each day). However, over the two days that the children ate the low energy density meals, their total two-day energy intake was 389 calories lower compared to the figure that was observed during the two days when high energy density foods were served. So, even three to five year olds will eat a given volume or weight of a food and if that food has a lower energy density they will eat fewer calories. Well, one could argue that two days isn't long enough so the team obtained access to data from a previous study where 658 subjects were given dietary advice to manage blood pressure which included dietary advice to increase intakes of fruits and vegetables over a six-month period.[14] Because these foods are high in water content but low in calories, it follows that these subjects were put on a lower energy density diet. Of course some embraced the fruit and vegetable advice more so than others, so it was possible to divide the subjects into three groups where the reductions in energy density were small, medium or large. Those who had the smallest decrease in their energy density showed a weight loss of 2.4 kilograms while those with the largest decrease in energy density had twice this weight loss (5.9 kilograms). So the evidence for longer term advantages of a low energy dense diet on weight loss greatly strengthens the case for this type of dietary advice. The final area of investigation that I want to draw on here is how portion size influences caloric intake when energy density is manipulated. Professor Rolls and her group devised four identical diets to cover a two-day period of study. The two extremes were a high energy density and a high portion size versus a low energy density and a low portion size. In between there was a reduced energy density with a high portion size, and a reduced portion size with a high energy density. Both portion size and energy density influenced caloric intake as predicted and the effects were additive. So a 25% decrease in portion size led to a 10% decrease in caloric intake, while a 25% increase in energy density led to a 24% increase in caloric intake.

Against all that background of research, Professor Rolls has published several diet books promoting the value of weight loss and weight maintenance through reductions in energy density. In *The Ultimate Volumetrics Diet*, Professor Rolls spells out the basic theory behind weight loss and maintenance by reducing energy density. First she prepares the diet plan with a series of questions to ascertain if the reader is really ready to make the long-term commitment to a diet. This reinforces what I said at the beginning of this chapter about the need to be sure that there are good grounds for losing weight and that now is the time to do it. She then tackles the important issue of a suitable target weight, not too ambitious but enough to be a significant long-term challenge. Physical activity is, as it always should be, an integral part of a weight loss programme and Professor Rolls gives good tips on the subject, but more of that in the third book which we will come to very shortly.

All of the foods and dishes in Professor Rolls's book are classified into caloric density categories (CD). In category CD1 are almost all fruits and non-starchy vegetables and broth-based soups. These are free to eat anytime but that doesn't mean you can eat dozens of apples at a sitting! CD2 is whole grain foods, lean meat, fish and poultry, legumes and low fat dairy products. These are to be eaten in reasonable portions. CD3 includes bread, desserts, fat-free baked snacks, cheese and higher fat meats and these are to be eaten through careful management of portions. Fried snacks, candy, cookies, nuts and fats are in CD4 and these require very careful management of both portion size and frequency. The book then takes the reader through breakfast, lunch, dinner, snacks and eating out and gives general guidelines and tips on how to achieve a lower caloric density choice for each meal. Then there is a four-week meal plan with advice for each day as to breakfast, lunch and evening meal amounting to 84 recommendations. The reader can pick and choose from within any of the meal categories according to their own personal tastes and preferences. Finally, there are over 170 individual recipes covering all meal categories.

Unlike most diet books, this one stands out a mile. It is written by a world-leading scientist and is based on really powerful science. It doesn't cut out any food and it doesn't advocate specific foods rich say in protein or fat. It doesn't promise a quick, easy and simple solution and it doesn't promise to help shed loads of pounds in no time at all. As a final salute to the power of caloric or energy density to manage weight, one can turn to no less an august organisation than the US Dietary Guidelines Advisory Committee who completed a detailed review of the literature in this field and concluded 'that strong and consistent evidence in adults indicate that dietary patterns relatively low in energy density improve weight loss and weight maintenance'.

The final book I will turn to is on physical activity and weight management, Professor James Hill of the University of Colorado Medical School is the lead author.[15] Much of the data in chapter seven originate from Professor Hill's lab and his accumulated experience in the field of physical activity and weight management led him and his colleagues to produce an excellent book entitled *The Step Diet*. The first stage in the Step Diet is to establish baseline measurements. This involves keeping a food diary for a week and wearing a pedometer for that week. A pedometer comes with the book. Although the focus of the book is based around how many steps per day you need to take, he recommends a food diary, not for counting calories, but to try to record your sense of overeating. As with the other authors of the books covered in this chapter Professor Hill and his co-authors recognise the huge role that passive eating plays in weight gain. So, the idea of the diary is to instil a discipline to avoid mindless eating. As with Brian Wansink, the authors also focus on this mindless additional 100 calories, which if sustained daily would lead to a five-pound gain in weight over a year. A critically important principle of this book is that you have to learn how to avoid weight gain before you start thinking about weight loss. The book therefore advocates small changes in lifestyle. Thus to stop gaining weight, the first small change is to increase the number of steps you take by 2,000. You should be able to achieve that in 20 minutes and you can do this all in one go or in two to three stages throughout the day. These additional 2,000 steps will equate to 100 calories. Having successfully incorporated an extra 2,000 steps into your daily routine, the next stage is to set your weight management goals. A 5% weight loss will be relatively easy whereas a 15% weight loss is a tougher goal so, sensibly, we might start with a 5% weight loss and having achieved that, consider further weight loss. The authors recommend a 12-week weight loss period. This is long enough to lose weight and reduce the adverse effects of excess fat but not so long as to grow weary of the small changes you are about to implement. From here on in, it's all about counting steps and not calories. The first table you turn to is to gauge how many steps you need to take to burn off one calorie. For me weighing 109 kilograms (240 pounds) and measuring 1.9 metres in height (six foot two inches)) it is 14 steps. These steps are referred to in the book as life steps. For my wife (120 pounds and five foot six) it is 29 steps per calorie. Bear in mind the physics here.

To move a heavy object takes more energy than to move a lighter object. The same is true of humans walking. But also remember that my stride is longer than my wife's so when we walk together and we both wear pedometers, she gets more steps from the walk than I do. The next stage is to calculate your resting metabolic rate, not in calories, but in steps. As was pointed out previously, your resting metabolic rate is the energy you expend to breath, filter blood in the kidneys, digest your food, maintain your brain power, pump blood around the body and so on. For me that works out at 27,400 steps per day and for my wife it is 34,600 steps per day based on a large table in the book. These are referred in the book as body steps since the number of steps corresponds to your body's resting metabolic rate. Remember, my wife needs more steps per calorie than I do. So, after you've increased your steps per day by 2,000 you record your total steps per day. If you engage in physical activity that does not involve steps such as swimming or cycling, there is a table for such activities in steps per minute for any given activity. So if you cycle to work for 15 minutes in each direction every day, you add 180 steps per minute for a male, which amounts to 5,400 steps. Once you have measured your average life steps, you first add this to your body steps, which are now your total daily steps from exercise and basal metabolic rate. You calculate what percentage of your total daily steps your life steps account for. Yesterday I played nine holes of golf and the total number of life steps I accumulated was 10,329. My body steps were 27,425 so my total daily steps yesterday was 37,754. Thus 10,329 is 27.4% of 37,754 so my physical activity yesterday was 27.4% of all the energy I expended. Now the day before, I spent all of it writing this book so my total daily steps was 3,065 and that equates to just 10% of my total energy as physical activity. On average, most people leading a sedentary lifestyle will burn off only 10% to 15% of their total daily energy expenditure as physical activity.

Now here is the crunch. Extensive data show that unless you average 25% of daily energy expenditure as physical activity you will not sustain weight loss. Once you have computed your baseline data and stopped any weight gain with your additional 2,000 steps per day, you are now ready for your 12-week programme of weight loss and this will involve both diet and physical activity. As regards diet, the advice in the book is simple: leave 25% of your food behind you. Brian Wansink favours 20% and he advocates that you don't put it on your plate bearing in mind that we eat with our eyes. Leaving 25% behind might provide in my view too big a temptation so I'd favour Wansink's view of simply plating out 20% less of everything except vegetables, which we should plate out 20% more of. That fits in with what Professor Rolls advises in decreasing our energy density. Each week, you increase your body steps by 500 such that by the end of 12 weeks you will have added another 6,000 steps to your count. Taking the additional 2,000 you added at the beginning, you have now increased your pre-diet steps by 8,000. An average middle-aged person leading a sedentary lifestyle will have about 4,000 steps, which will now become 12,000 steps per day. That will definitely exceed the threshold of 25% of daily energy expenditure to maintain weight loss. More is of course better but within reason because overdoing exercise can cause joint problems and eventually become boring. The more you can build your daily steps into your everyday routine, the more likely you are to maintain the increased activity. As was pointed out earlier, when you lose weight your basal metabolic rate will fall. So when you've lost weight, you multiply the pounds lost by eight to calculate your fall in resting metabolic rate and you convert that back to steps based on the tables linking height and weight to steps per calorie. You readjust your body steps downward by that amount and now set your goals based on that figure. It may seem complicated but *The Step Diet* takes you through it all with ease and plenty of examples.

Because the total daily steps figure can be long with five digits, the authors recommend that you divide this figure by 1,000. So if I had an average of 38,000 total daily steps, I can alter that to 38 mega steps per day, assuming I play nine holes of golf. If I sit in front of the computer all day it is down to 30 mega steps. This is really handy to understand the relationship of steps to food. A glass of wine for me is one mega step. A Chinese meal such as 24 ounces of chicken chow mein is 12 mega steps. In effect, this one dish equals my entire physical activity for the day. That surprises most people but my calculation is that this much chicken chow mein is 580 calories. If most people are at just 15% of energy in physical activity and their total daily calories are say 2,000, then they will expend no more than 300 calories, half the caloric value of a serving of chicken chow mein. Understanding food in steps is far better than in calories because we can easily understand steps and what to do about them.

Taking all three books into account, my advice on weight loss would be as follows:

- Have a check-up to ascertain whether or not you have adverse health consequences of overweight.
- Discuss the management of these problems with your doctor and even if you do lean toward drugs to manage conditions such as heart disease or high blood pressure, give weight loss a thought as an option.

- Don't take over-the-counter diet pills.
- Be aware that most dieters relapse within two years. Set realistic goals and keep a daily diary.
- Try to be aware of mindless eating so only serve yourself 80% of the non-vegetable component of the meal and increase the vegetable component by 20%.
- Try to eat more slowly and aim to finish when you are no longer hungry, not when you are full.
- Familiarise yourself with the concept of energy density and experiment with recipes, which have a low energy density.
- Always start your meal with the lowest energy dense foods such as salads or soups.
- Get yourself a pedometer and aim to have at least 10,000 steps daily on average, which means sedentary days have to be followed by quite active days.
- Build walking into your everyday life as much as possible.
- Anticipate setbacks and be prepared for them.

As Mary Pickford the Canadian actress and co-founder of United Artists Motion Studio said: 'You may have a fresh start any moment you choose, for this thing we call "failure" is not the falling down, but the staying down.' From the personal perspective we now move to conclude this book with two final chapters. The first looks at the national perspective and at the opportunities and limits to what might be achieved but it doesn't actually give opinions on what should be done. That is for the final chapter.

CHAPTER THIRTEEN

Weight Management:
The National Perspective

In science, there are core tenets that are beyond dispute. Water boils at 100 degrees centigrade, the sun rises in the east, not all swans are white and grass is green. As regards the regulation of body weight, there is also a fundamental tenet: the continued consumption of calories above daily caloric requirements will lead to obesity. But beyond that, differences exist as to the main causes of energy imbalance and consequently, differences exist as to what should be done to redress these imbalances in energy in versus energy out equations. The philosopher of science Thomas Kuhn argued that scientists generally defend theories or schools of thought rather than challenge them and that the only way that a school of thought might change is when some revolutionary scientific facts emerge. An example of revolutionary science would be the experiment completed by the Medical Research Council in the UK which showed beyond any shadow of doubt, under stringent experimental conditions, that additional folic acid over and above what is usually available from the diet, halved the recurrence of neural tube defects among women who previously had given birth to children with spina bifida, the most common of such neural tube birth defects.[1] Once the revolution came, the new school of thought was formed and now the details could be worked out: exactly how much folic acid in the diet and exactly what level of folic acid in the blood was optimal? Could one get enough folic acid through normal dietary means? Which is the better measure of habitual folic acid intake: the level in blood plasma or the levels in red blood cells?

Beyond the basic tenet of obesity that weight gain is caused by excessive caloric consumption, there is no certainty. Some experts are drawn to the role of processed foods, others to poor socio-economic status, others to snacking, to fast food, to exercise, to sugar-sweetened beverages and so on. Once a scientist becomes a card-carrying member of some given school of thought, all his or her efforts are directed, not at refuting this concept, but defending and promoting it.

We have previously encountered Daniel Kahneman's concept that the mind operates in two systems: System 1 operating automatically and System 2 involving 'effortful mental activities'. System 2 might be the driving force for someone deciding to focus their interests in obesity around socio-economic status, sugar-sweetened beverages, fast food, fructose or whatever. But after that System 2 decision, all subsequent data and scientific findings are adopted or rejected within System 1, primarily on the basis of whether they support the position arrived at initially in System 2. He makes a telling point when he states: 'Contrary to the rules of philosophers of science, who advise testing hypotheses by trying to refute them, people (and scientists, quite often) seek data that are likely to be compatible with the beliefs they currently hold.'[2] In the interests of transparency, let me state my position based on my System 2 analysis of obesity. I believe it to be extremely complex, multi-faceted and not at all subject to simple solutions. Thus when I see for example a paper explaining why television advertising causes obesity in children, my System 1 tends to instantly dismiss it as overly simplistic. Were it one element of a larger multi-faceted analysis I could live with it. It is thus important for readers of this book to understand that the pursuit of solutions to obesity are driven by scientific views that are not always derived from comprehensive and detailed analytical processes. Once an 'expert' goes public on his or her opinion on one particular policy strategy as a means of combating obesity, there is no turning back. As Abraham Maslow's stated in his book *The Psychology of Science*: 'If all you have is a hammer, everything looks like a nail.'

Against that concept of inherent bias in thinking among all scientists in highly complex areas such as obesity, let's now look at some possible approaches to combat this dreadful public health scourge of obesity. To do so, I choose to draw on a report of the Nuffield Council on Bioethics, an internationally acclaimed, independent body in the UK, funded by the Wellcome Trust and the Medical Research Council. The report is entitled *Public Health: Ethical Issues*.[3] A key part of this report is what is referred to as the 'intervention ladder', comprising eight levels of approach to tackling public health issues. In the words of the report: 'The further up the ladder the state goes, the stronger the evidence has to be.' In this instance, evidence exists in two dimensions. The first dimension relates to evidence that the proposed intervention is based on firm scientific principles. If there is compelling evidence that some particular factor is independently linked to a risk of weight gain in children, then the first dimension of evidence is met. The second dimension embraces evidence that, in fact, the proposed intervention to redress this imbalance in this causative risk factor would be successful. So, it's not enough to say A causes B. We must show that by changing C, we can change B and, by implication, A. Often we have some evidence on the A–B link but not on the C–A link. This chapter is in fact a prelude to the final chapter where I outline my personal views on how best to tackle obesity. Rather than offering solutions, it forces a detailed consideration of their respective challenges.

Step 1. 'Do Nothing or Simply Monitor the Current Situation'

Whether we like it or not, great swathes of the world are sufficiently concerned about their body weight that they are doing something to manage it, according to one large Nielsen poll.[4] Given the global scale of the problem, and given the very considerable level of public concern about body weight and health, it would be unthinkable to 'Do nothing or simply monitor the current situation'. Monitoring is widespread in most countries and the plethora of statistics on national obesity prevalence is testimony to that fact. Our scientific journals are awash with the findings of these research programmes. This monitoring should not be ad hoc or part of some wider data collection system. Rather it should be centrally coordinated and targeted. If childhood obesity is of primary concern, a programme to monitor the condition in children should be implemented annually.

There are, however, in my opinion glaring omissions from the routine collection of data. Imagine initiating a complex, well-conceived and well-funded campaign on diet, physical activity and obesity where a large population of the target affected audience did not recognise themselves as relevant to the campaign. This, I'm afraid, happens all the time since the proportion of overweight and obese subjects who do not recognise they have a problem is very significant. Large US national surveys covering all age groups show that a great many people who are defined by weight and height as overweight and obese, dispute this. They simply deny they are carrying excessive weight.[5] And this is a finding that is found the world over. A staggering 80% of boys and girls, who are overweight, believe their weight is healthy. Just about half of obese boys and about two thirds of obese girls believe their weight is normal. Against that background, ask yourself how useful weight control campaigns are. Whether it be taxation, banning, limiting, pricing, advertising or labelling mediated, all such programmes will be left with a problem: large numbers of the intended audience don't feel that such an intervention applies to them. It is someone else's problem. In the vast majority of countries that aspire to manage obesity, this deficit is not properly addressed and thus by and large, interventions programmes start off with one hand tied behind their backs. It takes time by researchers and considerable ongoing investment by funding agencies to tackle this root problem so it tends to get ignored, ensuring of course that all subsequent public health interventions are fundamentally flawed. In all subsequent steps, assume that this basic need of communication on the true impact of people's actual BMI is in place and having a very positive effect.

Step 2. 'Provide Information'

My colleagues very often tick this box quite quickly and point to food labels, guideline daily amounts, local and national educational campaigns, communicative tools such as the food pyramid and such like. I don't accept this as adequate. Let me take as a comparative example television advertisements here in Ireland released by the Road Safety Authority to reduce the annual death and injury rate from road traffic accidents. Almost daily and often several times a day we see such ads. An accident and emergency physician in clinical garb and with the signatory stethoscope around his neck tells us about the horrific injuries he sees through seat belt non-use or misuse. This ad campaign also warns car drivers about care around motorcyclist and cyclists, about walking on the roads especially at night, about the use of social drugs and of smartphones while driving. All of these are powerful images, and are broadcast several times a night, every night of the week. No one would dispute their need and value given that 166 people on Irish roads in 2015. Ireland isn't alone in this television road safety campaign. Most other countries are on par in both the scale of the problem and its address by way of television ad campaigns. But I can count on one seriously mutilated hand the number of adverts I ever see on any national television service for the treatment and management of obesity, excluding of course the many ads for whacky ideas on food and health or equally whacky ads on maintaining a healthy body weight. Road traffic death and injuries carry a public dread that overweight does not. Hence it is more politically important. So when my friends battle about the relevant advantage of front, side or back of nutrition labelling, I think that they are kidding themselves. Important as such information may be, head-on, properly coordinated television, radio and social media communication campaigns on nutrition and health are essential if we are to successfully address the problem, or even make inroads into it.

Step 3. Enable Choice

Individuals alone can make changes to their diet and by definition their choice of food and their choice of physical activity level. So how can the state make sure that the choices people are offered will include ones that will enable better weight management through diet and physical activity? The state may make and repair roads and bicycle lanes, it can build parks and install fitness areas in them, it can create pedestrian areas in built-up zones, it can create sports facilities and it can do many things to improve recreational exercise. But it doesn't make food nor does it process, distribute or cook our foods. Farmers provide fresh food and the food industry provides prepared, packaged and processed foods. So it is up to the food industry to provide choices. You can buy sugar-sweetened beverages or sugar-free beverages. You can buy full fat or low fat or no fat milk. You can buy meat or fish or poultry and you can buy lean or fatty meat. So the food industry has provided choice by and large. In some cases, options are not really possible. Thus a fish and chip shop has little option but to provide traditional fish and chips and there is really no consumer demand for any deviation from that since that is what people expect from a fish and chip meal. However, in both the food industry and the catering sector, food portion sizes can be modified so that one has the option to buy smaller serving sizes. Failure to deliver options to choose smaller portions is therefore a significant barrier to the enabling of consumer choice. The state can contribute by facilitating or regulating the entire food chain such that choice is enabled for the consumer. Choice means making a decision, hopefully informed, as to two or more food options thus improving diet quality. The McKinsey Global Institute's report on obesity ranks portion control as the top intervention in terms of lowest cost and highest impact, reducing the adverse effects of obesity.[6] It addresses the issue of portion control to food producers, restaurateurs and work canteens. It recognises a frequently ignored dimension to action by industry to change existing practices. Some might praise food companies for reducing portion sizes but they might be criticised from two constituencies. One might be shareholders who see the competition failing to act likewise and thus gaining a competitive edge in the market. The other is the consumer who might believe that a smaller serving of French fries in the work canteen should cost less. In reality, the cost of the food on the plate is minimal compared to the main costs of the food service operation such as rent, property and water taxes, insurance, equipment depreciation, heating, lighting and salaries. So, some intervention by the state can help the market to adapt uniformly to reduced portion sizes in a manner, which is fair to consumer and producer. In this way, better food choice might be enabled.

Here I have two major problems with McKinsey. By my calculation about 60% of calories purchased by Irish adults in supermarkets come from fresh foods (meat, poultry, fish, eggs, milk, cheese, butter, bread, fruit, vegetables etc.). All are fresh, loose or pre-packed for convenience. About 25% of our national food is from the food service sector (restaurants, pubs, chip shops etc) and about 15% from processed, pre-prepared foods where portion control might be applied. But who decides how much butter I put on my bread or how much cheese I put into my sandwich? Who stands in the kitchen to regulate the portions selected by the family from a plate of roast beef, a bowl of roast potatoes, a bowl of vegetables and jugs of gravy, not to mention the glasses of wine or soft drinks consumed at a family meal? Who decides how much porridge I should put in my bowl in the morning or how much milk and sugar I add to the porridge? Portion control, like so many attractive solutions to the obesity crisis is not as straightforward as many make it out to be, including the learned folk at McKinsey. However, the bottom line is that in the enabling of choice between healthier and less healthy foods or higher and lower serving sizes, any help from any quarter, which fosters better choice, is welcome. But as always, policies have to be realistic. Food portion control is only partially managed by the vendor.

A second issue I have with this assumption that reduced portion size by vendors is necessarily as good as it's made out to be is that very little data exist to cover the issue of frequency of intake. You can reduce portion size of pizzas down to a glowingly low level but that will have no impact if two such pizzas are purchased over time rather than one. An extensive review of the literature would suggest that the growth in BMI over time is indeed associated with portion size but is even more strongly related to frequency of food ingestion.[7] So which is better to regulate or try to change: serving size or frequency of consumption? And who has the Solomon-like wisdom to know the difference?

Step 4: Guide Choices through Changing the Default Policy

If we were successful in Step 2 and 3 we would have both an enlightened and motivated consumer with access to a food chain that offers ample choice in pursuing a healthy diet and managing body weight. We can now go one step further but we have reached a rung in the ladder where we are beginning to diminish choice. Fast food outlets such as Burger King, McDonald's and Wendy's have dropped sugary drinks as an automatic inclusion in its children's meal offers.[8] Children can still be served soft drinks, but they will have to be purchased separately from the combo meals designed for them. The kid's meal pack will now contain milk, chocolate milk, apple juice or water. Remember the work of Brian Wansink with mindless eating? By introducing a step, which for a millisecond moved from mindless to mindful eating, better food intake control was achieved. This approach of default positioning of diet soft drinks offers the consumer the chance to move from a mindless to a mindful choice. Could this be extended to all food outlets, fast or otherwise, where the default becomes the smaller portion and that the consumer must ask for the larger portion? Could it work in restaurants, bars and canteens? There cannot be a default in the kitchen other than we encourage smaller plates. But in the food service sector, changes to healthier choices as the default are possible, subject to the issues raised in the preceding section on competition and consumer expectations of food pricing. However, caution is needed when deciding to introduce a new, healthier default option. Both involve school meals and sugar. In 2011–12, chocolate flavoured milk was by far the most popular milk among the overall flavoured milk available in 11 Oregon elementary schools.[9] A decision was reached to ban chocolate flavoured milk as part of a sugar reduction programme. The consequences were simple. Total milk intake fell by 10% and 7% of students stopped taking school meals. Overall, regular milk sales rose by 100% but waste of this milk was up by 24%. Was this a success? Another example includes a study of the effect of a fat intervention programme over several years in certain schools taking part in the National School Lunch Intervention Programme.[10] The aim was to reduce total fat to 30% of calories and saturated fats to 10% of calories. A total of 76 schools were included in the intervention arm and 22 schools where no intervention was implemented served as a control group. As schools met the total fat and saturated intervention, they fell down on sugar which increased wherever fat was lowered. The authors conclude: 'The existence of a fat-sugar "see-saw" makes it important to emphasize substitutions of fat and saturated fat with starches and fiber in school lunches.' So, yes it's a good thing to challenge the default position but as my carpenter father used to say: 'Measure twice, cut once!'

Step 5. Guide Choice through Incentives

In many countries, it is possible to purchase a bicycle from your salary before tax, which means that you have a discount on the purchase of the bicycle equal to the top rate of tax you pay. This is a real incentive to increase physical activity. Schemes such as this can be quite easily policed but once you introduce incentives, particularly fiscal incentives, the opportunity for fraud increases. If the state, employers and vendors did not strictly police the pre-tax bicycle scheme, the bicycle market would be dominated by fraud. Health insurance companies offer incentives toward health screening but they rarely modify their costs to the consumer based on any health index and certainly not on any diet-related health index. Subsidies to join gyms might be considered, as might subsidies to join weight control programmes. In fact, in many countries, a sales tax applies to such services, which immediately introduces a disincentive. It is often suggested that government subsidies on low fat, low energy dense foods such as fruits, vegetables and pulses would help. But how would this operate? One option might be to refund the vendor 10% of the price of the product passing on that saving to consumers. How would this be policed? How would it operate in large supermarket chains, local corner groceries, petrol or gas stations or stalls in airports and railways and of course for street vendors and farmers' markets? And what if the price of the product falls to the vendor such as when market prices for fruit and vegetables fall, perhaps due to good growing conditions? How can we be sure that the 10% subsidy is being passed on in full to the consumer? How would restaurant and canteen companies cope? Then we would have to ask the question: could a 10% reduction in the price of fresh fruit and vegetables cause a shift in consumption of other foods and if so, among those who did manage to change consumption, how can we measure its contribution to obesity? If convenience is more important than price, will a 10% change in cost matter? Regrettably, the devil is in the detail. This does not mean that society should not seek incentives to change eating habits but it does mean, yet again, that what often seems a simple solution is often not so. We could also look at removing disincentives to healthy eating and healthy lifestyle choices.

Step 6: Guide Choice through Disincentives

We now move to the deliberate disincentive to make healthy choices and here we are definitely into the territory of limiting freedom. The most widely talked about disincentive in food choice is that relating to the introduction of taxes on foods deemed to be contributors to obesity. Because we are at the near upper end of the intervention ladder, we must now probe forensically into the benefit and risk of taxing particular foods.

As a general rule, one would rightly start off with a series of questions with an expectation that detailed consideration had been given to each and every aspect of the issue in question and that a policy maker would shape policy based on a comprehensive review of the matter. These are the questions to which I would seek an answer:

- On what basis have you decided to seek a tax on this food rather than others and has your econometric model been applied to a range of foods to inform your present particular choice?
- If we introduce a tax as you recommend, what end points would you use to measure success, and over what time period, and do you have, at present, baseline data with which to gauge progress?
- Have you considered any adverse outcomes of this proposed tax and, if so, what are they? Do you intend to monitor these possible adverse effects and if so by what criteria and with reference to which baseline data?

Now all of this may sound pretty 'spoil sportish' in that there may be a public head of steam to push for some given tax. However, it doesn't seem unreasonable to ask the hard questions and to entertain this forensic analysis.

I'd like to consider the global favourite for food taxation namely sugar-sweetened beverages (SSBs) and I will use data from the National Adult Nutrition Survey here in Ireland to address the issue.[11] Let's start off with the first question above. When we look at the data, we see that the category 'table sugar, syrups, jams and marmalade' accounts for 12% of average adult caloric intake. Next comes the category 'biscuits, cakes, pastries and buns' at 11%, then SSBs at 8% and then 'chocolate confectionery' at 7%. Have all these foods been the subject of an econometric model? The answer is no because taxing SSBs is a global fashion, a meme as previously described. Next let us look at the impact of SSBs alone. Among males aged 18–64, 43% of the population are regular consumers and among females the comparable figure is 31%. That averages

37%, which means that 63% of the population, of whatever weight they might be, will never be hit by this tax and will never benefit from this initiative. The advocates point out that among teens, the figures are much higher but this is not a society dominated by teens. It can also be argued that a focus on taxing SSBs will help move a whole generation from a high level of consumption of these products. But none of this negates the fact that among 18 to 60 year olds, this strategy simply ignores 63% of the population. Maybe a biscuit cake and bun tax or a chocolate tax or a table sugar and jam tax would target the adults more. But such taxes are not on the table because they are not part of the global fashion of SSB taxation. SSBs are identified with corporate whipping boys such as Coca-Cola and corporate culpability for obesity rides high on the populist agenda.

According to an econometric model applied to the Irish market, a 10% tax on SSBs would lead to a reduction in energy intake of 2.1 calories per day with a 1.2% reduction in the number of persons who are obese.[12] Or would it? As we saw in earlier chapters the human body weight regulates its energy balance very well. Whether the body can actually detect changes as small as 2.1 calories per day is questionable on two levels. Firstly, it implies a great level of precision on the true caloric content of foods and since the caloric value of foods is computed from its composition (carbohydrate, protein, fat, alcohol and to the nearest decimal point), it's difficult to be confident about such small values. Secondly, we know that there are major levels of energy under-reporting (up to 50%) and this is not necessarily built into the econometric model. Indeed, if true caloric intakes were higher because of this phenomenon of under-reporting, then we might be talking a little higher than 1.2 calories per day and we might reach a quantitative deficit that we could have increased confidence in. The problem here is that as the deficit in caloric intake grows due to the increasing restriction of sugar intake, the more likely we will record energy compensation. In other words, as we take calories out of a person's diet through the restriction of the availability of sugar, and as we do so surreptitiously and by stealth, the person is very likely to defend their daily caloric requirement through the consumption of foods other than those targeted for their sugar content. The net effect is a rise in the total fat intake. This sugar–fat seesaw has been observed year on year, continent by continent, study after study. Indeed, intervention studies that surreptitiously remove sugar calories, inevitably lead to energy compensation and to a rise in percentage energy from fat, as outlined earlier. SSBs are believed to be immune from this energy compensation because they are in liquid form and so immune to energy compensation but the evidence is limited. Now at present, the media have sugar as a popular toxin with fat released, as it were, on parole for rehabilitation. Thus to summarise: if we want to tax a particular food, we need to come forward with strong evidence that the choice of that particular food or group of foods is fully justified based on a comprehensive risk analysis. In general, that isn't done.

To return now to the second of the questions posed, one would want to know the end points that would be used to determine efficacy of a policy of SSBs taxation. Would it be a reduction in the number of persons purchasing SSB products? Would it be a reduction in overall percentage energy from sugar with (or without) a comparable rise in percentage energy from starchy foods or fatty foods? Would it be an overall reduction in energy intake? Would it involve a change in average body weight? Of course all of the above questions can only apply to those who consume SSB products and have no bearing on the majority of us who don't consume SSBs. The challenge I see here is that such end points are never spelled out and if they were, we would need both a baseline measure before the introduction of a tax, followed by several further measures over a pre-defined time period, to assess the efficacy of the taxation strategy.

As regards adverse effects, which are raised in the third question above, we can argue that a risk exists that as sugar is shed, fat is taken on board as just outlined. But there is one other downside to the taxing of foods in that the taxation process may end up being regressive. What that means is that it will cause greater hardship among those who are socially deprived. One study here in Ireland showed very clearly that a tax on 'bad foods' would hurt the economically disadvantaged but that a subsidy of 'good foods' would negate this and be budget neutral.[13] The first problem here would be defining 'good' and 'bad foods' within the context of overall 'good' or 'bad' daily or weekly diets. The second problem is operating the subsidy as discussed earlier in this chapter and avoiding fraud. In the US the Women, Infants and Children Program uses vouchers, which are distributed to the socially disadvantaged and even then, fraud is widespread.[14] All in all, taxing foods is a minefield of contentious arguments with advocates frequently opting for a very narrow perspective toward a simple solution.

Step 7: Restrict Choice and Step 8: Eliminate Choice

This is unexplored territory for public health nutrition. Restricting choice might be to prohibit the sale of French fries in work and school canteens to three days per week, or it might be the banning of snack vending machines from schools and hospitals. Eliminating choice might be to ban the farming of sugar! If taxation of foods is a challenge, then, the restriction or elimination of foods hits directly at the rights of humans to select their own foods and there is no doubt that these steps will make lawyers, especially constitutional lawyers, very rich.

And so we move to the final chapter, a personal vision on what needs to be done to tackle the obesity issue.

CHAPTER FOURTEEN

The Way Forward

And so we come to the final part of this book. Having studied the problem, putative causes and consequences, and the frameworks and players involved, we meet the big question: how do we move the issue forward? I write this section alone and not as an expert member of an appropriate committee so I don't have any committee colleagues to challenge me with alternate thoughts and interpretations, new data, queries and corrections. What I write would, in effect, be my opening gambit if I were ever asked to sit on an expert committee on diet, physical inactivity and weight management. Let me start with the reality of where we are now.

The Reality We Face

The reality of the problem we face is best covered by two quotations from a UK government Foresight report on obesity issued in 2010. The report entitled *Tackling Obesities: Future Choices* remains, in my view, the most sensible, analytical, balanced and comprehensive review of the problems of obesity.[1] As regards the possible causes of obesity, the report points out:

> What quickly becomes apparent to anyone who examines the body of evidence from several different disciplinary sources is that the answers are neither straightforward nor, as is popularly supposed, necessarily known. Although a great deal of research has been done into the problem, much of the evidence is not integrated.

The key criticism here is that absolute lack of integration in national strategies to resolve the obesity level. That lack of integration as to possible causes is matched by a similar deficit in tackling the causes of obesity. The report notes:

The complexity and interrelationships of the obesity system described in this report make a compelling case for the futility of isolated initiatives. Focusing heavily on one element of the system is unlikely to bring about the scale of change required. There are as yet no concerted strategies or policy models that adequately address the problem.

Thus, in this chapter my approach will be toward the minimisation of single-issue approaches and to maximise integrated approaches. In the last *Lancet* series on obesity, recognition was given of the need for 'top down' and 'bottom up' approaches to the resolution of the obesity and physical inactivity challenges.[2] For the purposes of this book, I would prefer to use alternate terms that are more easily understood by the consumer. For 'top down' I would prefer the 'regulatory environment'. For 'bottom up', I would prefer 'community led approaches'. In either case, it is important to be crystal clear as to how the national landscape would change as a result of either or both intervention approaches. For some, the dream is that of a physically fit, obesity-free society. That in my view is a pipe dream. We might reduce the average BMI and we might reduce the percentage of people above some high level of BMI. In advance, I do not know what figures to put on these targets but some ballpark evidence-based target would have to be established. For me, BMI is a problem, not because it requires people to wear XXL clothes or to be sylph-like on the beach. For me it is a problem because higher BMI and a sedentary lifestyle lead to serious risk factors for chronic diseases, primarily high blood pressure and impaired glucose metabolism. Thus if I wanted to dabble in the metrics of public health intervention targets, I'd first be looking for baseline blood pressure and fasting blood glucose values and I'd be setting SMART-based targets to reduce their national prevalence (I will explain SMART in ensuing sections). The main effect of this is that I no longer bother people about weight, which as we have seen, they can misunderstand and I would not be chasing any embarrassment factor. Programmes to know your blood pressure and to know your glucose tolerance are without stigmatisation, are attainable with minimal visits to the health services and can be targeted through any one or all of three strategies: diet, physical activity and drugs. I would, in addition to this screening for risk factors, be seriously promoting physical activity and would have a very soft watch on weight. This I know is not a popular view and avoids the obesity elephant in the room. But the cast iron statistics are that treated obesity returns at an alarming rate and the elephant tends to linger. Success with physical activity, blood pressure and diabetes management could be linked to some form of fiscal incentives for participants – a reduction in private health premiums, reduced costs to participate in physical activity such as with gyms or swimming pools and so on. Notwithstanding what I'd like to see happen in any national campaign, reduction in BMI is the target of almost all programmes that are based in the regulatory environment or in a community-based approach, a review of which now follows.

The Regulatory Environment

In the realm of road safety, we are required by law to have a seat belt fitted in our cars and all passengers are required to wear them. Moreover, we may not drive a car with a certain level of alcoholic drink taken, we may not drive while using narcotics and we must obey speed limits and the rules of the road. With food, we can do what we like. However, there are rules that govern food safety and authenticity, and relevant authorities police these laws. Public health, steeped in the tradition of banning, prohibiting, curbing, restricting, licensing and so on, turns to such traditional solutions when faced with the public health issue of obesity. These then become the 'isolated initiatives' referred to in the UK Foresight report on obesity. We have looked at one such example, sugar taxation, previously, so let's look at some others.

Labelling: For years, manufacturers of foods have been required to add material to food labels from pack size to ingredient details. In nearly every jurisdiction now, some form of nutritional labelling is required. For the average consumer, this poses a challenge. How do you read the small print that necessarily characterises nutrition labels with limited pack space and make a universal judgement on the nutritional value of one food over another? To overcome this and make life easy, one approach has been to create a formula into which all the food's nutritional ingredients are entered and which, at the end, determines whether the food gets a red, amber or green 'light' placed on the front of the pack.[3] Now in choosing a tinned soup or whatever, the red light version is going to attract less interest than a green light version, among nutrition conscious consumers. Of course, among consumers concerned with value for money, price is all-important. Many such 'traffic light' systems exist and each has its own set of champions, to some extent in competition with one another. There are criticisms of this simple approach in its own right and criticisms of labelling in general. As regards the latter, labelling doesn't really work with fresh foods (never labelled) or with the 25% plus of our calories consumed in food service sectors from street vendors to fine dining to pub food to work canteens. Secondly, labelling all foods according to a single formula makes it difficult for manufacturers to set either internal or sectoral cut-off points for nutritional composition for specific food categories. For example, to improve the nutritional value of an average serving of a pizza will require a different set of targets to the optimal nutritional reformulation of say breakfast cereals or frozen desserts. Whatever the outcome, any labelling that helps consumers make intelligent and useful food choices is to be welcomed.

Calories on menus: This is an extension of food labelling in that it brings us directly into the restaurant, pub, fast food outlet, the school or work cafeteria or anywhere where consumers make food choices for direct and immediate consumption.[4] Central systems exist in some regions to allow caterers use online systems to obtain data on calorie values for their dishes. So a consumer can look both at price and calories when choosing starters, main courses and desserts. Some argue that this simply leads to certain consumers looking for the maximum number of calories for the least price. Others argue that nobody cares about calories when they go out to eat. However, surely this helps those who are trying to manage their weight? Yes there are problems for self-service menus and yes there are challenges to fine dining establishments who like to change their menus frequently. But for the weight conscious, a level of consciousness that we are trying to promote in society, this must be helpful.

Portion size: This is a complex example I'll use to illustrate the 'regulatory environment' approach to the issues of overweight. The McKinsey report highlighted portion size as the public health initiative that would produce the greatest bang for our buck in tackling obesity. I have previously highlighted some of the challenges to portion control, not least when food is prepared at home or at self-service food outlets. A detailed systematic review of this topic by a high level expert group concluded thus:

> This review found that people consistently consume more food and drink when offered larger-sized portions, packages or tableware than when offered smaller-sized versions. This suggests that policies and practices that successfully reduce the size, availability and appeal of larger-sized portions, packages, individual units and tableware can contribute to meaningful reductions in the quantities of food (including non-alcoholic beverages) people select and consume in the immediate and short term. However, it is uncertain whether reducing portions at the smaller end of the size range can be as effective in reducing food consumption as reductions at the larger end of the range.[5]

Again, these data support some element of control of portion size in the regulation of caloric intake. The big question is how do you regulate this? Labelling might be one approach. Thus for a pizza, irrespective of its size, a portion could be promoted using some text or graphic approach. But pizzas tend to be eaten freshly prepared either at home or in some area of the food service sector so can we realistically expect this to work on large pizzas? Could we enact legislation to set a legal limit on the sale of pizzas above a certain size? Would this really work, if as previously mentioned that frequency of consumption is as big a determinant of food intake as portion selection? Could food retailers be forced to always offer both a normal and a 'starter' portion size on their menu and what data do we have that both food service sector outlets and consumers would accept this? Some of these could of course be considered in any bottom up approach within overall nutrition education of the general public. All in all, however, each of these show that what seem obvious and simple moves in the realm of the regulatory environment, are not without significant reality checks. The biggest regulatory challenge of all is the 'food industry' to which we now turn our attention.

The food industry: The food industry is seen as the consummate enemy of those who would like to reshape our present lifestyles to one where caloric intake and caloric output are at all times perfectly balanced. Many international and governmental agencies go to great lengths to ensure that big industry does not have the opportunity to exert undue influence in their decision-making processes and, in fairness, that is exactly what consumers want and deserve. However, unlike the tobacco, alcohol and firearms industries, getting rid of the food industry is simply not an option. It hasn't been so for millennia as has been previously pointed out in earlier chapters. The big companies remain the villains for several reasons. They are globally recognised through their brands. They play a global role in sports sponsorship for the World Cup to the Olympic Games. They absolutely dominate the food advertising industry. They are the ones who innovate and come up with new, tasty products and new solutions to health challenges. They, and they alone, represent the food chain when dialogue is made with national or international agencies in either food safety or nutrition. But they still make up a small part of the global food chain. Most of our dietary cholesterol intake comes from eggs. Name a global figure in egg production? Name a global figure in salad sales or bread sales or the sales of trout, steak, shellfish, cabbage, chicken, potato or freshly baked cakes? You probably can't. But you can name global food companies who sell breakfast cereals, ice cream, pizzas, biscuits, savoury snacks, sugar-sweetened beverages, yoghurts, margarines, sweets, chocolate and so on. And now we have two choices: live with them in a regulated environment or live without them. Suppose I had some magic wand given to me by some wandering spirit and with this wand I could eliminate the global food sector. Consumer demand for some foods might fall but the present role of the Danones, the Mars, the Nestlé's, the Coca-Colas and the like would simply be replaced by a new tier as the sector reshuffled itself. So we have no choice but to sit down with the existing multinational food companies and work out targets. This isn't helped by sensationalist articles in some medical journals linking high level scientists who advise their government on nutrition issues, with research funds received from the food industry.[6] The climate change players can develop bipartite solutions. Why can't the food sector? The food industry will have to abide by initiatives that are evidence-based and will also have to live with initiatives that are somewhat weak on evidence but which seem to the majority, worthy of pursuit. From this writer's current perspective this is not possible at present. There is little or no global dialogue between industry and governments in tackling obesity with some obvious exceptions and presently, even the most respected research scientists with the highest research outputs are considered persona non-grata with high level agencies if they are even part funded by industry.

The Community-Based Approach

I want to begin with what looks like a community-based approach but which was a top down approach. In 1992, the Singaporean government recorded a level of overweight and obesity in schoolchildren of 14%. They set about introducing the Trim and Fit programme (TAF). All students from primary level to pre-university level were targeted and, in fact, the selection criterion for involvement in the programme was a body weight 120% of the ideal weight for a given age group. This was not a programme that parents and children opted to join: this was compulsory. In addition to the normal level of physical activity, those who were entered into this programme had to engage in 1.5 hours of additional supervised physical activity sessions that included all forms of physical activity including sports activity. The children had to set aside special time for these activities; coming earlier to school or leaving later to fulfil the requirements of the programme. In addition to physical activity programmes, the children had intense nutrition counselling and were given food coupons which rationed the amount of calories they could get from school canteens. The coupons linked to calorie allowance to the degree of overweight. Above 160% of the ideal body weight, the children were referred to a special health promotion board with more intense counselling, and ultimately to paediatricians. The level of childhood obesity fell to 9.8% within one decade. Understandably, the level of stigmatisation of the children obliged to take part in this programme was unprecedented. In 2005, researchers from Singapore noted a six-fold rise in eating disorders, specifically anorexia nervosa and bulimia. Two years later, this TAF programme was abandoned and replaced by one aimed at all school children. Very few would hold that this austere programme, effectively an intrusion into the human rights of children and their families, should be a model for top down obesity approaches. It should be noted that the driving force behind all of this was the demand of the Singaporean military for fit, active, slim and health recruits!

Turning now to a true bottom up approach, the example I've taken was started in France and was the brainchild of an endocrinologist. It was a school-based intervention programme in two towns in northern France (Fleurbaix and Laventie) with two comparable towns acting as controls, starting in 1992.[7] The town councils gave full support to the programme and built new physical activity facilities as well as facilitating the training of schoolteachers in nutrition to help deliver the programme. Two full-time dietitians were appointed to manage the programme, and the help of general practitioners, pharmacists, shopkeepers and sport and cultural organisations were enlisted. In just over a decade, this community-based, concerted action led to a reduction in BMI among boys with a value of 15.6 compared to a baseline value of 16.7 in the control towns. For girls, the respective values were 15.7 and 16.4. It is important to note that the effects only became evident after eight years of constant reinforcement of the programme's objectives with full community support. The authors noted:

> However, it was apparent that interventions targeting schools alone were not sufficient, and that progress was only made when the mobilization of the population became more generalised at community level and involved schools, pre-schools, local sports and parents associations, catering structures, health professionals, elected representatives, and local stakeholders from the public and private sectors.

This study gave rise to a comparable initiative globally entitled EPODE (Ensemble Prévenons l'Obesité Des Enfants – Together Let's Prevent Childhood

Obesity).[8] There are four pillars in the EPODE methodology: (1) political commitment, which is central to the initiative; (2) resources which directly fund central support services and local implementation; (3) support services with an emphasis on social marketing to provide evidence based communication programmes; and (4) programmes that are using evidence at all times to inform the delivery of the programme and to evaluate its impact. EPODE is but one example. Others exist but they never hit the headlines. Without community-based activities, however anonymous, no real progress will ever be made in tackling physical inactivity and obesity.

Sustaining Structures

In the UK Foresight report on obesity, the conclusion writes of the 'futility of isolated initiatives'. In reality, nothing happens without a plan and no plan is successful if it doesn't embrace all forces for change. It is this writer's view that unless, and until, governments establish independent agencies with a sole remit to tackle obesity and physical inactivity, progress will be ad hoc and painfully slow. Most civilised countries have independent food safety authorities, independent road safety authorities and comparable authorities for all sorts of social good. Why not independent agencies properly funded and charged with long-term management of this enormous public health problem? This is the organisation to integrate the many isolated initiatives, to provide baseline data, to set out SMART objectives – objectives that are highly specific, measurable, attainable, realistic and time-bound. This would be a well-funded organisation. In order to get the metrics right – set them straight. Let me return to the preface where mention was made of a $20 trillion cost over the lifetime of all US youths who retained that obesity into adulthood. My simple calculations equate this with both the construction costs and 40-year lifetime maintenance costs of about 30–40 US nuclear submarines of the Virginia class. That's a lot of money. My guess is that an agency in the US comparable to the FDA that would tackle top down and bottom up approaches to obesity would cost over 40 years about as much as one submarine. No matter what way you do the maths, the bottom line is that permanent, independent, well funded agencies are within most national budgets. The resources are there. It's just the will that is lacking. No dough, no go! Will it ever happen? I hope so.

Notes

Preface

1   World Health Organization (2009) *Global Health Risks: Mortality and Burden of Disease Attributable to Selected Major Risks*. Geneva: WHO.

2   Brookings Institute. Available at: brookings.edu/~/media/events/2015/05/12-economic-costs-of-obesity/0512-obesity-presentation-v6-rm.pdf (Accessed October 2015).

3   Stuckler, D. and Nestle, M. (2012) 'Big food, food systems, and global health'. *PLOS Medicine*, 9 (6).

4   Obama, M. 'Feeding the planet, energy for life: highlights from the First Lady's visit to Milan Expo'. Posted by Deb Eschemeyer, Executive Director of Let's Move! Available at: letsmove.gov (Accessed September 2015).

5   Sullivan, G. 'The blind spot in the anti-soda crusade', Healthy Living. *The Huffington Post*, 2015. Available at: huffingtonpost.com/news/bloomberg-soda-ban (Accessed September 2015).

Chapter One: Ever Seen a Fat Fox?

1   Pagel, M. (2012) *Wired for Culture: The Natural History of Human Cooperation*. London: Allen Lane.

2   Dawkins, R. (2014) *The Selfish Gene*. Oxford: Oxford University Press.

3   Harari, Y. N. (2014) *Sapiens: A Brief History of Human Kind*. London: Harvill Secker.

4   Armstrong, K. (2009) *The Case for God: What Religion Really Means*. London: The Bodley Head.

5   Slovic, P. (2000) *The Perception of Risk*. London: Earthscan.

6   McKinsey Global Institute (2014) *Overcoming Obesity: An Initial Economic Analysis*. Available at: mckinsey.com/insights/economic_studies/how_the_world_could_better_fight_obesity (Accessed September 2015).

7   Ibid.

8   Dolan, P. (2014) *Finding Happiness by Design: Finding Pleasure and Purpose in Everyday Life*. London: Allen Lane.

9   Kahneman, D. (2011) *Thinking Fast and Slow*. London: Penguin Group.

10 Chabris, C. F. and Simons, D. J. (2010) *The Invisible Gorilla: And Other Ways Our Intuitions Deceive Us*. New York: Crown.

11 Ritzer, G. (1993) *The McDonaldization of Society*. Thousand Oaks: Pine Forge Press.

12 Dolan, P. and Galizzi, M. M. (2014) *Because I'm Worth It: A Lab-Field Experiment on the Spillover Effects of Incentives in Health*. Center for Economic Performance Discussion Paper 1286. Available at: cep.lse.ac.uk/pubs/download/dp1286.pdf.

13 Syrad, H., Falconer, C., Cooke, L., Saxena, S., Kessel, A. S., Viner, R., Kinra, S. and Wardle, J. (2015) '"Health and happiness is more important than weight": a qualitative investigation of the views of parents receiving written feedback on their child's weight as part of the National Child Measurement Programme'. *Journal of Human Nutrition and Dietetics*, 28: 47–55.

Chapter Two: Measurements and Metrics

1 Ramsay, M. A. E. (2006) 'John Snow, MD: anaesthetist to the Queen of England and pioneer epidemiologist'. *Baylor University Medical Center Proceedings*, 19: 24–8.

2 Gey, K. F. (1990) 'The antioxidant hypothesis of cardiovascular disease: epidemiology and mechanisms'. *Biochemical Society Transactions*, 18: 1041–5.

3 The Alpha-Tocopherol Beta Carotene Cancer Prevention Study Group (1994) 'The effect of vitamin E and beta carotene on the incidence of lung cancer and other cancers in male smokers'. *The New England Journal of Medicine*, 330:1029–35.

4 Sackett, C. S. and Schenning, S. (2002) 'The age-related eye disease study: the results of the clinical trial'. *Insight*, 27: 5–7.

5 Obican, S. G., Finnell, R. H., Mills, J. L., Shaw, G. M. and Scialli, A. R. (2010) 'Folic acid in early pregnancy: a public health success story'. *The FASEB Journal*, 24: 4167–74.

6 Mensink, R. P. and Katan, M. B. (1990) 'Effect of dietary trans fatty acids on high-density and low-density lipoprotein cholesterol levels in healthy subjects'. *New England Medical Journal*, 323: 439–45.

7 Association of Life Insurance Medical Directors (1912) *Medico-Actuarial Mortality Investigations*. New York: Association of Life Insurance Medical Directors and Actuarial Society of America.

8 Metropolitan Life Insurance Company (1942) 'Ideal weights for men'. *Statistical Bulletin (Metropolitan Life Insurance Company)*, 23: 6–8.

9 Metropolitan Life Insurance Company (1959) 'New weight standards for men and women'. *Statistical Bulletin (Metropolitan Life Insurance Company)*, 40:1–4.

10 Metropolitan Life Insurance Company (1983) 'Metropolitan height and weight tables'. *Statistical Bulletin (Metropolitan Life Insurance Company*, 64:1–19.

11 Keys, A., Fidanza, F., Karvonen, M. J., Kimura, N. and Taylor, H. L. (1972) 'Indices of relative weight and obesity'. *Journal of Chronic Diseases*, 25: 329–43.

12 National Institute of Health (1985) 'Health implications of obesity'. Available at: consensus.nih.gov/1985/1985Obesity049html.htm (Accessed October 2015).

13 World Health Organization (1998) *Obesity: Preventing and Managing the Global Epidemic*. Geneva: WHO.

14 Abel, R. C., Somers, V. K., Sierra-Johnson, J., Thomas, R. J. et al. (2008) 'Accuracy of body mass index to diagnose obesity in the US adult population'. *International Journal of Obesity*, 32: 959–66.

15   Garn, S. M., Leonard, W. R. and Hawthorn, V. M. (1956) 'Three limitations of the body mass index'. *American Journal of Clinical Nutrition*, 44: 996–7.

16   Royal College of Physicians of London Working Party on Obesity (1983) 'Report on obesity'. *Journal of the Royal College of Physicians of London*, 17: 3–58.

17   Andres, R., Elahi, D., Tobin, J. D., Muller, D. C. et al. (1985) 'Impact of age on weight goals'. *Annals of Internal Medicine*, 103:1030–3.

18   Childers, D. K. and Allison, D. B. (2010) 'The obesity paradox: a parsimonious explanation for relations among obesity, mortality rate, and aging'. *International Journal of Obesity*, 34: 1231–8.

19   Flegal, K. M., Kit, B. M., Orpana, H. and Graubard, B. I. (2013) 'Association of all-cause mortality with overweight and obesity using standard body mass index categories: a systematic review and meta-analysis. *Journal of the American Medical Association*, 309: 71–82.

20   Hughes, V. (2013) 'The big fat truth: more and more studies show that being overweight does not always shorten life – but some public-health researchers would rather not talk about them'. *Nature*, 497: 428–30.

21   Jackson, C., Yeh, H. C., Szklo, M. and Hu, F. B. (2013) 'Body mass index and all-cause mortality in US adults with and without diabetes'. *Journal of General Internal Medecine*, 29: 25–33.

22   Murakami, K. and Livingstone, M. B. (2015) 'Prevalence and characteristics of mis-reporting of energy intake in US adults: NHANES 2003–2012'. *British Journal of Nutrition*, 24:1–10.

23   Mossavar-Rahmani, Y., Tinker, L. F., Huang, Y., Neuhouser, M. L., McCann, S. E., Seguin, R. A., Vitolins, M. Z., Curb, J. D. and Prentice, R. L. (2013) 'Factors relating to eating style, social desirability, body image and eating meals at home increase the precision of calibration equations correcting self-report measures of diet using recovery biomarkers: findings from the Women's Health Initiative'. *Nutrition Journal*, 12: 63–77.

24   Gibney M. J., Walsh, M., Brennan, L., Roche, H. M., German, B. and van Ommen, B. (2005) 'Metabolomics in human nutrition: opportunities and challenges'. *American Journal of Clinical Nutrition*, 82: 497–503.

Chapter Three: Human Obesity: Old and New

1   Kessler, D. A. (2009) *The End of Overeating: Taking Control of Our Insatiable Appetite.* London: Penguin Books, 3.

2   Conrad, N. J. (2009) 'A female figurine from the basal Aurigaician of Hohle Fels cave in southwest Germany'. *Nature*, 445: 248–52.

3   Foxcroft, L. (2011) *Calories and Corsets: A History of Dieting Over 2,000 Years.* London: Profile Books, 14.

4   Haslam, D. (2007) 'Obesity: a medical history'. *Obesity Review*, 8: 31–6.

5   Columella, L. (1485) *De Re Rustica.* Dehli: Gyan Books, 15.

6   Cornaro, L., Addison, J., Bacon, F. and Temple, W. (1903) *The Art of Living Long: A New and Improved English Version of the Old Treatise.* London: Bibliolife, 41.

7   Short, T. (1727) *A Discourse Concerning the Causes and Effects of Corpulent: Together with the Method for Its Prevention and Cure.* London: J. Robert, cited in L. Foxcroft, (2011) *Calories and Corsets*, 67.

8   Wadd, W. (1816) *Cursory Remarks on Corpulence, or, Obesity Considered as a Disease: With a Critical Examination of Ancient and Modern Opinions, Relative to Its Causes and Cure.* London: Smith and Davy, 3.

9   Symonds, B. (2010) 'Reprints and reflections: the influence of overweight and underweight on vitality'. *International Journal of Epidemiology*, 39: 951–7.

10   Komlos, J. and Brabec, M. (2010) *The Trend of Mean BMI Values of US Adults, Birth Cohorts 1882–1986 Indicates That the Obesity Epidemic Began Earlier than Hitherto Thought.* National Bureau of Economic Research. Available at: nber.org/papers/w15862 (Accessed September 2015).

11   Costa, D. and Steckel, R. H. (1997) 'Long-term trends in health, welfare and economic growth in the United States', in Steckle, R. H. and Floud, R. (eds) *Health and Welfare during Industrialization.* Chicago: University of Chicago Press.

12   Olsen, L. W., Baker, J. L., Holst, C. and Sørensen, T. I. (2006) 'Birth cohort effect on the obesity epidemic in Denmark'. *Epidemiology*, 17: 292–5.

13   National Taskforce on Obesity (2005) *Obesity: The Policy Challenges: The Report of the National Taskforce on Obesity.* Dublin: The Department of Health. Available at: hse.ie/eng/health/child/healthyeating/taskforceonobesity (Accessed October 2015).

14   Testimony before the Subcommittee on Competition, Infrastructure, and Foreign Commerce Committee on Commerce, Science, and Transportation United States Senate: "The Growing Epidemic of Childhood Obesity". Statement of Richard H. Carmona. Surgeon General. Available at: surgeongeneral.gov/news/testimony/childobesity03022004.html (Accessed September 2015).

15   Olds, T., Maher, C., Zumin, S., Péneau, S., Lioret, S., Castetbon, K., Bellisle, de Wilde, J., Hohepa, M., Maddison, R. et al. (2011) 'Evidence that the prevalence of childhood overweight is plateauing: data from nine countries'. *International Journal of Pediatric Obesity*, 6: 342–60.

16   Ogden, C. A., Carroll, M. D., Kiy, B. K. and Flegal, K. M. (2014) 'Prevalence of childhood and adult obesity in the United States'. *JAMA*, 311: 806–14.

17   Rokholm, B., Baker, J. L. and Sørensen, T. I. (2010) 'The levelling off of the obesity epidemic since the year 1999 – a review of evidence and perspectives'. *Obesity Review*, 11: 835–46.

Chapter Four: The Human Food Chain

1   Pollan, M. (2008) *In Defense of Food: An Eater's Manifesto.* New York: The Penguin Press, 149–50.

2   Nestle, M. (2010) 'How ultra-processed foods are killing us'. *The Atlantic*, 4 November. Available at: theatlantic.com/health/archive/2010/11/how-ultra-processed-foods-are-killing-us/65614. (Accessed October 2015).

3   Lustig, R. (2013) *Fat Chance: The Bitter Truth about Sugar.* London: Fourth Estate, 207–8.

4   Wrangham, R. (2009) *Catching Fire: How Cooking Made Us Human.* London: Profile Books.

5   Koebnick, C., Strassner, C., Hoffmann, I. and Leitzmann, C. (1999) 'Consequences of a long-term raw food diet on body weight and menstruation: results of a questionnaire survey'. *Annals of Nutrition and Metabolism*, 43: 69–79.

6   Fontana, L., Shew, J. L., Holloszy, J. O. and Villareal, D. T. (2005) 'Low bone mass in subjects on a long-term raw vegetarian diet'. *Archives of Internal Medicine*, 165: 684–9.

7   Cunnane, S. C. *Survival of the Fattest: The Key to Human Brain Evolution*.

8   Pagel, M. (2012) *Wired for Culture: The Natural History of Human Cooperation*. London: Allen Lane.

9   Cunnane, S. C. (2006) *Survival of the Fattest: The Key to Human Brain Evolution*. Singapore: World Scientific Publishing.

10 The Whaleback Shell Midden State Historic Site has a website outlining the story of these oysters. Accessible at: damariscottariver.org/trail/whaleback-shell-midden-state-historic-site (Accessed September 2015).

11 Fernández-Armesto, F. (2001) *Food: A History*. London: Macmillan.

12 Harlan, J. (1992) *Crops and Man*, 2nd Edition. Madison: American Society of Agronomy-Crop Science Society of America. Cited by Fernández-Armesto, F. (2001) *Food: A History*. London: Macmillan, 94.

13 Diamond, J. (1987) 'The worst mistake in the history of the human race'. *Discover*, May. Available at: discovermagazine.com/1987/may/02-the-worst-mistake-in-the-history-of-the-human-race (Accessed September 2015).

14 Ibid.

15 Ibid.

16 *Genesis* 3: 17–19.

17 Armelagos, G. J. (1984) Preface to the 2013 edition of Cohen, M. N. and Armelagos, G. J. (eds) *Paleopathology at the Origins of Agriculture*. Orlando: Academic Press.

18 McGovern, P. E., Zhang, J., Tang, J., Zhang, Z., Hall, G. R., Moreau, R. A., Nuñez, A., Butrym, E. D., Richards, M. P., Wang, C. S. et al. (2004) 'Fermented beverages of pre- and proto-historic China'. *Proceedings of the National Academy of Sciences*, 1011: 7593–8.

19 Toussaint-Samat, M. (2008) *History of Food*. Oxford: Blackwell Publishing.

20 Galloway, J. N., Leach, A. M., Bleeker, A. and Erisman, J. W. (2013) 'A chronology of human understanding of the nitrogen cycle'. *Philosophical Transactions of the Royal Society of London. Series B, Biological Sciences*, 368: 1–11.

21 Freidberg, S. (2009) *Fresh: A Perishable History*. London: Belknap Press.

22 Fried, S. (2011) *Appetite for America: Fred Harvey and the Business of Civilizing the Wild West – One Meal at a Time*. New York: Bantam Books.

Chapter Five: The Fashion of Culpable Calories

1   Skiadas, P. K. and Lascaratos, J. G. (2001) 'Dietetics in ancient Greek philosophy: Plato's concepts of healthy diet'. *European Journal of Clinical Nutrition*, 55: 532–7.

2   Vafeiadou, K., Weech, M., Altowaijri, H., Todd, S., Yaqoob, P., Jackson, K. G. and Lovegrove, J. A. (2015) 'Replacement of saturated with unsaturated fats had no impact on vascular function but beneficial effects on lipid biomarkers, E-selectin, and blood pressure: results from the randomized, controlled dietary Intervention and vascular function (DIVAS) study'. *American Journal of Clinical Nutrition*, 102: 40–8.

3   Reidlinger, D. P., Darzi, J., Hall, W. L., Seed, P. T., Chowienczyk, P. J. and Sanders, T. A. (2015) 'Cardiovascular disease risk reduction study (CRESSIDA) investigators. How

effective are current dietary guidelines for cardiovascular disease prevention in healthy middle-aged and older men and women? A randomized controlled trial'. *American Journal of Clinical Nutrition*, 101: 922–30.

4   Vigarello, G. (2013) *The Metamorphoses of Fat: A History of Obesity*. New York: Columbia University Press.

5   McCarrison, R. (1921) *Studies in Deficiency Disease*. London: Hodder & Stoughton.

6   Yudkin, J. (1986) *Pure, White and Deadly: The New Facts about the Sugar You Eat as a Cause of Heart Disease, Diabetes and Other Killers*. London: Viking Press.

7   Lustig, R. (2013) *Fat Chance: The Bitter Truth about Sugar*. London: Fourth Estate.

8   Hannah, A. C. (1997) 'The world sugar market and reform'. *FAO Corporate Depository*. Available at: fao.org/docrep/005/x0513e/x0513e09.htm (Accessed September 2015).

9   Tappy, L. and Egli, L. (2008) 'Metabolism of nutritive sweeteners in humans', in Rippe, J. M. (ed.) *Fructose, High Fructose Corn Syrup, Sucrose and Health*. London: Humana Press, 35–50.

10   Moeller, S. M., Fryhofer, S. A., Osbahr, A. J. 3rd, Robinowitz, C. B. and Council on Science and Public Health, American Medical Association (2009) 'The effects of high fructose syrup'. *The Journal of the American College of Nutrition*, 28: 619–26.

11   American Dietetic Association (2004) 'Position of the American Dietetic Association: use of nutritive and nonnutritive sweeteners'. *Journal of the American Dietetic Association*, 104: 255–75.

12   Marriot, P., Fink, C. J. and Krakower, T. (2008) 'Worldwide consumption of sweeteners and recent trends', in Rippe (ed.) *Fructose, High Fructose Corn Syrup, Sucrose and Health*: 87–11.

13   These data are available at: iuna.net (Accessed October 2015).

14   Danziger, S., Levav, J. and Avnaim-Pessoa, L. (2011) 'Extraneous factors in judicial decisions'. *Proceedings of the National Academy of Sciences*, 108: 6889–92.

15   Hall, K. D., Bemis, T., Brychta, R., Chen, K. Y., Courville, A., Crayner, E. C., Goodwin, S., Guo, J., Howard, L., Knuth, N. D. et al. (2015) 'Calorie for calorie, dietary fat restriction results in more body fat loss than carbohydrate restriction in people with obesity'. *Cell Metabolism*, 22: 427–36.

16   Taubes, G. (2007) *Good Calories, Bad Calories*. New York: Alfred A Knopf.

17   Jebb, S. A., Prentice, A. M., Goldberg, G. R., Murgatroyd, P. R., Black, A. E. and Coward, W. A. (1996) 'Changes in macronutrient balance during over- and underfeeding assessed by 12-d continuous whole-body calorimetry'. *American Journal of Clinical Nutrition*, 64: 259-66.

18   Markey, O., Le Jeune, J. and Lovegrove, J. A. (2015) 'Energy compensation following consumption of sugar-reduced products: a randomized controlled trial'. *European Journal of Nutrition*, published online September 2015.

19   Chen, L., Appel, L. J., Loria, C., Lin, P. H., Champagne, C. M., Elmer, P. J., Ard, J. D., Mitchell, D., Batch, B. C., Svetkey, L. P. et al. (2009) 'Reduction in consumption of sugar-sweetened beverages is associated with weight loss: the PREMIER trial1–3'. *American Journal of Clinical Nutrition*, 89: 299–306.

20   Sørensen, L. B., Vasilaras, L. H., Astrup, A. and Raben, A. (2014) 'Sucrose compared with artificial sweeteners: a clinical intervention study of effects on energy intake, appetite, and energy expenditure after 10 wk of supplementation in overweight subjects'. *American Journal of Clinical Nutrition*, 100: 36–45.

21 American Heart Association and American Diabetes Association (2012) 'Nonnutritive sweeteners: current use and health perspectives'. *Diabetes Care*, 35: 1798–1808.

22 Sadler, M. J., McNulty, H. and Gibson, S. (2015) 'Sugar–fat seesaw: a systematic review of the evidence'. *Critical Reviews in Food Science and Nutrition* 55: 338–56.

23 Cullen, M., Nolan, J., Cullen, M., Moloney, M., Kearney, J., Lambe, J. and Gibney, M. J. (2004) 'Effect of high levels of intense sweetener intake in insulin dependent diabetics on the ratio of dietary sugar to fat: a case-control study'. *European Journal of Clinical Nutrition*, 58: 1336–41.

24 Scientific Advisory Committee on Nutrition (2015) *Carbohydrates and Health*. London: HMSO.

25 Augustin, L. S., Kendall, C. W., Jenkins, D. J., Willett, W. C., Astrup, A., Barclay, A. W., Björck, Brand-Miller, J. C., Brighenti, F., Buyken, A. E., Ceriello, A. et al. (2015) 'A glycemic index, glycemic load and glycemic response: an International Scientific Consensus Summit from the International Carbohydrate Quality Consortium (ICQC)'. *Nutrition, Metabolism and Cardiovascular Disease*, 25: 795–81.

Chapter Six: The Nature versus Nurture Debate

1   Wadd, W. (1816) *Cursory Remarks on Corpulence, or, Obesity Considered as a Disease: With a Critical Examination of Ancient and Modern Opinions, Relative to Its Causes and Cure.* London: Smith and Davy.

2   Short, T. (1727) *A Discourse Concerning the Causes and Effects of Corpulency: Together with the Method for Its Prevention and Cure.* London: J. Robert.

3   Clague, A., Thomas, A. (2002) 'Neonatal biochemical screening for disease'. *Clinica Chimica Acta*, 315: 99–110.

4   Friedman, J. M., Halaas, J. L. (1998) 'Leptin and the regulation of body weight in mammals'. *Nature*, 395: 763–70.

5   Farooqi, I. S. and O'Rahilly, S. (2014) '20 years of leptin: human disorders of leptin action'. *Journal of Endocrinology*, 223: T63–T70.

6   Angulo, M. A., Butler, M. G. and Cataletto, M. E. (2015) 'Prader-Willi syndrome: a review of clinical, genetic, and endocrine findings'. *Journal of Endocrinological Investigation*, 38 (12): 1249–63.7 Wardle, J., Carnell, S., Haworth, C. M. and Plomin, R. (2008) 'Evidence for a strong genetic influence on childhood adiposity despite the force of the obesogenic environment'. *American Journal of Clinical Nutrition*, 87: 398–404.

8   Dubois, L., Ohm Kyvik, K., Girard, M., Tatone-Tokuda, F., Pérusse, D., Hjelmborg, J., Skytthe, A., Rasmussen, F., Wright, M. J. and Lichtenstein, P. (2012) 'Genetic and environmental contributions to weight, height, and BMI from birth to 19 years of age: an international study of over 12,000 twin pairs'. *PLOS One*, 7: e30153.

9   Stunkard, A. J., Harris, J. R., Pedersen, N. L. and McClearn, G. E. (1990) 'The body mass index of twins reared apart'. *The New England Journal of Medicine*, 322: 1483–7.

10 Sørensen, T. I. and Stunkard, A. J. (1993) 'Does obesity run in families because of genes? An adoption study using silhouettes as a measure of obesity'. *Acta Psychiatrica Scandinavica*, 370: 67–72.

11 Bouchard, C., Tremblay, A., Després, J. P., Nadeau, A., Lupien, P. J., Thériault, G., Dussault, J., Moorjani, S., Pinault, S. and Fournier, G. (1990) 'The response to long-term overfeeding in identical twins'. *The New England Journal of Medicine*, 322: 1477–82.

12 Bouchard, C., Tremblay, A., Després, J. P., Thériault, G., Nadeau, A., Lupien, P. J., Moorjani, S., Prud'homme, D. and Fournier, G. (1994) 'The response to exercise with constant energy intake in identical twins'. *Obesity Research*, 2: 400–10.

13 Llewellyn, C. and Wardle, J. (2015) 'Behavioral susceptibility to obesity: gene-environment interplay in the development of weight'. *Physiology & Behavior*, 2015 Jul 10. pii: S0031-9384(15)30022-6.

Chapter Seven: Regulating Food Intake

1 Fisher, C. and Scott, T. R. (1972) *Food Flavours: Biology and Chemistry*. Cambridge: Royal Society of Chemistry paperbacks.

2 Piqueras-Fiszman, B. and Spence, C. (2014) 'Colour, pleasantness and consumption behaviour within a meal'. *Appetite*, 75: 165–72.

3 Morewedge, C. K., Huh, Y. E. and Vosgreau, J. (2010) 'Thought for food: imagined consumption reduces actual consumption'. *Science*, 330:1530–3.

4 Chambers, A. P., Sandoval, D. A. and Seeley, R. J. (2013) 'Central nervous system integration of satiety signals'. *Current Biology*, 23: 379–88.

5 Brunstrom, J. M. (2014) 'Mind over platter: pre-meal planning and the control of meal size in humans'. *International Journal of Obesity*, 38: S9–S12.

6 Coll, A. P., Farooqi, I. S. and O'Rahilly, S. (2007) 'The hormonal control of food intake'. *Cell*, 1229: 251–62.

7 Carvalho, G. B. and Damasio, A. (2013) 'The nature of feelings: evolutionary and neurobiological origins'. *Nature Reviews Neuroscience*, 14: 143–52.

8 Craig, A. D. (2002) 'How do you feel? Interoception: the sense of the physiological condition of the body'. *Nature Reviews Neurobiology*, 3: 655–66.

9 Berthoud, H. R. and Morrison, C. (2008) 'The brain, appetite and obesity'. *Annual Review of Psychology*, 259: 55–92.

10 Mela, D. J. (1999) 'Food choice and intake: the human factor'. *Proceedings of the Nutrition Society*, 58: 513–21.

11 Forde, C. G., Almiron-Roig, E. and Brunstrom, J. M. (2015) 'Expected satiety: application to weight management and understanding energy selection in humans'. *Current Obesity Reports*, 4: 131–40.

12 Brunstrom, J. M. (2011) 'The control of meal size in human subjects: a role for expected satiety, expected satiation and premeal planning'. *Proceedings of the Nutrition Society*, 70: 155–61.

13 Forde, C. G., Almiron-Roig, E., Brunstrom, J. M. (2015) 'Expected satiety: application to weight management and understanding energy selection in humans'. *Current Obesity Report*, 4 (1): 131–40.

14 Wansink, B., Painter, J. E. and North, J. (2005) 'Bottomless bowls: why visual cues of portion size may influence intake'. *Obesity Research*, 13: 93–100.

15 Fay, S. H., Ferriday, D., Hinton, E. C., Shakeshaft, G., Rogers, P. J. and Brunstrom, J. M. (2011) 'What determines real-world meal size? Evidence for pre-meal planning.' *Appetite*, 6: 284–9.
16 Schachter, S. (1968) 'Obesity and eating: the internal and external cues differentially affect the eating behaviour of obese and normal subjects'. *Science*, 161: 751–6.
17 Carnell, S. and Wardle, J. (2008) 'Appetite and adiposity in children: evidence for a behavioural susceptibility theory of obesity'. *American Journal of Clinical Nutrition*, 88: 22–9.
18 Cassady, B. A., Considine, R. V. and Mattes, R. D. (2012) 'Beverage consumption, appetite, and energy intake: what did you expect?' *American Journal of Clinical Nutrition*, 95: 587–93.
19 Llewelyn, H., van Jaarsveld, C., Johnson, L., Carnell, S. F. and Wardle, J. (2010) 'Nature and nurture in infant appetite: analysis of the Gemini twin birth cohort.' *American Journal of Clinical Nutrition*, 91: 1172–9.
20 Cooke, L., Carnell, S., and Wardle, J. (2006) 'Food neophobia and mealtime food consumption in 4–5 year old children.' *International Journal of Behavioral Nutrition and Physical Activity*, 6: 3–14.
21 Carnell, S., Haworth, C. M. A., Plomin, R., and Wardle, J. (2008) 'Genetic influences on appetite in children.' *International Journal of Obesity*, 32: 1468–73.
22 Karra, E., O'Daly, O. G., Choudhury, A. I., Yousseif, A., Millership, S., Neary, M. T., Scott, W. R., Chandarana, K., Manning, S., Hess, M. E. et al. (2013) 'A link between FTO, ghrelin, and impaired brain food-cue responsivity'. *The Journal of Clinical Investigation*, 123: 3539–52.
23 Wardle, J., Carnell, S., Haworth, C. M. A., Farooqi, S., O'Rahilly, S., Plomin, R. (2008) 'Obesity Associated Genetic Variation in FTO is associated with diminished satiety'. *The Journal of Clinical Endocrinology and Metabolism*, 93: 3640–3.

Chapter Eight: Fitness and Fatness

1 Kohl, H. W. 3rd, Craig, C. L., Lambert, E. V., Inoue, S., Alkandari, J. R., Leetongin, G., Kahlmeier, S. and *Lancet* Physical Activity Series Working Group (2012) 'The pandemic of physical inactivity: global action for public health. *Lancet*, 380: 294–305.
2 FBI budget request for fiscal year 2015. Available at: fbi.gov/news/testimony/fbi-budget-request-for-fiscal-year-2015 (Accessed September 2015).
3 'The black budget.' *The Washington Post*. Available at: washingtonpost.com/wp-srv/special/national/black-budget/ (Accessed September 2015).
4 US Department of Homeland Security (2015) 'Budget-in-brief: fiscal year 2015'. Available at: dhs.gov/sites/default/files/publications/FY15BIB.pdf (Accessed September 2015).
5 World Health Organization (2009) *Global Health Risks: Mortality and Burden of Disease Attributable to Selected Major Risks*. Geneva: WHO.
6 Swinburn, B., Sacks, G. and Ravussin, E. (2009) 'Increased food energy supply is more than sufficient to explain the US epidemic of obesity'. *American Journal of Clinical Nutrition*, 90: 1453–6.
7 Church, T. S., Thomas, D. M., Tudor-Locke, C., Katzmarzyk, P. T., Earnest, C. P. et al. (2011) 'Trends over 5 decades in US occupation-related physical activity and their associations with obesity.' *PLoS One*, 6 (5): e19657.

8   Hall, K. D., Guo, J., Dore, M. and Chow, C. C. (1995) 'The progressive increase of food waste in America and its environmental impact'. *PLOS One*, 4 (11): e7940.

9   Prentice, A. M. and Jebb, S. A. (1995) 'Obesity in Britain: gluttony or sloth?'. *BMJ*, 311: 437–9.

10   Mira, L., Katz, M. L., Amy, K., Ferketich, A. K., Broder-Oldach, B., Harley, A., Reiter, P. L., Paskett, E. D. and Bloomfield, C. D. (2012) 'Physical activity among Amish and non-Amish adults living in Ohio Appalachia'. *Journal of Community Health*, 37: 434–40.

11   Ekelund, U., Ward, H. A., Norat, T., Luan, J., May, A. M., Weiderpass, E., Sharp, S. J., Overvad, K., Østergaard, J. N., Tjønneland, A. et al. (2015) 'Physical activity and all-cause mortality across levels of overall and abdominal adiposity in European men and women: the European Prospective Investigation into Cancer and Nutrition Study (EPIC)'. *American Journal of Clinical Nutrition*, 103 (3): 613–21.

12   Ptdirect 'Tools for personal training success'. Available at: ptdirect.com/training-design/exercise-behaviour-and-adherence/attendance-adherence-drop-out-and-retention-patterns-of-gym-members (Accessed October 2015).

13   Church, T. S., LaMonte, M. J., Barlow, C. E. and Blair, S. N. (2005) 'Cardiorespiratory fitness and body mass index as predictors of cardiovascular disease mortality among men with diabetes'. *Archives of Internal Medicine*, 16: 2114–20.

14   Hu, G., Tuomilehto, J., Silventoinen, K., Barengo, N. and Jousilahti, P. (2004) 'Joint effects of physical activity, body mass index, waist circumference and waist-to-hip ratio with the risk of cardiovascular disease among middle-aged Finnish men and women'. *European Heart Journal*, 25: 2212–19.

15   Li, T. Y., Rana, J. S., Manson, J. E., Willett, W. C., Stampfer, M. J., Colditz, G. A., Rexrode, K. M. and Hu, F. B. (2006) 'Obesity as compared with physical activity in predicting risk of coronary heart disease in women'. *Circulation*, 113: 499–506.

16   Barry, V. W., Baruth, M., Beets, M. W., Durstine, J. L., Liu, J. and Blair, S. N. (2014) 'Fitness vs. fatness on all-cause mortality: a meta-analysis'. *Progress in Cardiovascular Diseases*, 56: 382–90.

17   Centers for Disease Control and Prevention (2011) *Strategies to Prevent Obesity and Other Chronic Diseases: The CDC Guide to Strategies to Increase Physical Activity in the Community*. Atlanta: US Department of Health and Human Services.

18   Villablanca, P. A., Alegria, J. R., Mookadam, F., Holmes, D. R. Jr, Wright, R. S. and Levine, J. A. (2015) 'Non-exercise activity thermogenesis in obesity management'. *Mayo Clinic Proceedings*, 90: 509–9.

19   Levine, J. A., Schleusner, S. J. and Jensen, M. D. (2000) 'Energy expenditure of non-exercise activity'. *American Journal of Clinical Nutrition*, 72: 1451–4.

20   Levine, J. A., Eberhardt, N. L. and Jensen, M. D. (2000) 'Role of non-exercise activity thermogenesis in resistance to fat gain in humans'. *Science*, 283: 212–14.

21   Koepp, G. A., Manohar, C. U., McCrady-Spitzer, S. K., Ben-Ner, A., Hamann, D. J., Runge, C. F., James, A et al. (2013) 'Treadmill desks a 1-year prospective trial'. *Obesity*, 21: 705–11.

Chapter Nine: A Miscellany of Matters

1   BBC (2011–2012) 'The Nine Months that Made You'. Available at: https://www.youtube .com/watch?v=4g9HUtT3baw (Accessed October 2015).

2   United States Department of Agriculture (2015) 'Household food security in the United States in 2014'. Available at: ers.usda.gov/media/1896841/err194.pdf (Accessed October 2015).

3   Park, K., Kersey, M., Geppert, J., Story, M., Cutts, D. and Himes, J. H. (2009) 'Household food insecurity is a risk factor for iron-deficiency anaemia in a multi-ethnic, low-income sample of infants and toddlers'. *Public Health Nutrition*, 12 (11): 2120–8.

4   Berti, C., Biesalski, H. K., Gärtner, R., Lapillonne, A., Pietrzik, K., Poston, L., Redman, C., Koletzko, B. and Cetin, I. (2011) 'Micronutrients in pregnancy: current knowledge and unresolved questions'. *Clinical Nutrition*, 30 (6): 689–701.

5   Darmon, N. and Drewnowski, A. (2015) 'Contribution of food prices and diet cost to socioeconomic disparities in diet quality and health: a systematic review and analysis'. *Nutrition Reviews*, 73: 643–60.

6   Rayner, J. (2013) *A Greedy Man in a Hungry World: How (Almost) Everything You Thought You Knew about Food Is Wrong*. London: Collins.

7   Wang, F., Zhang, L., Zhang, Y., Zhang, B., He, Y., Xie, S., Li, M., Miao, X., Chan, E. Y., Tang, J. L., Wong, M. C., Li, Z., Yu, I. T. and Tse, L. A. (2014) 'Meta-analysis on night shift work and risk of metabolic syndrome'. *Obesity Reviews*, 15: 709–20.

8   Institute for the Study of Labor (2007) *Obesity, Unhappiness, and the Challenges of Affluence: Themes and Evidence*. Bonn: IZA. Available at: http://ftp.iza.org/dp2717.pdf (Accessed October 2015).

9   Coffin, C. S. and Shaffer, E. A. (2006) 'The hot air and cold facts of dietary fibre'. *Canadian Journal of Gastroenterology*, 20 (4): 255–6.

10   Irish Universities Nutrition Alliance. Available at: www.iuna.net (Accessed October 2015).

11   Rosenbaum, M., Knight, R. and Leibel, R. L. (2015) 'The gut microbiota in human energy homeostasis and obesity'. *Trends in Endocrinology and Metabolism*, 26 (9): 493–501.

12   Hanage, W. P. (2014) 'Microbiology: microbiome science needs a healthy dose of scepticism'. *Nature*, 512 (7514): 247–8.

13   American Psychiatric Association. Available at: dsm5.org/Pages/Default.aspx (Accessed October 2015).

14   Stice, E., Burger, K. S. and Yokum, S. (2013) 'Relative ability of fat and sugar tastes to activate reward, gustatory, and somatosensory regions'. *American Journal of Clinical Nutrition*, 98 (6): 1377–84.

15   Ziauddeen, H., Farooqi, I. S. and Fletcher, P. C. (2012) 'Obesity and the brain: how convincing is the addiction model?'. *Nature Reviews Neuroscience*, 13 (4): 279–86.

16   Cunnane, S. C. (2006) *Survival of the Fattest: The Key to Human Brain Evolution*. Singapore: World Scientific Publishing, 63.

17   Avena, N. M., Rada, P., Moise, N. and Hoebel, B. G. (2006) 'Sucrose sham feeding on a binge schedule releases accumbens dopamine repeatedly and eliminates the acetylcholine satiety response'. *Neuroscience*, 139 (3): 813–20.

18 Pursey, K. M., Stanwell, P., Gearhardt, A. N., Collins, C. E. and Burrows, T. L. (2014) 'The prevalence of food addiction as assessed by the Yale Food Addiction Scale: a systematic review'. *Nutrients*, 6 (10): 4552–90.

19 Lent, M. R., Eichen, D. M., Goldbacher, E., Wadden, T. A. and Foster, G. D. (2014) 'Relationship of food addiction to weight loss and attrition during obesity treatment'. *Obesity*, 22 (1): 52–5.

20 Carlsson, L. M., Peltonen, M., Ahlin, S., Anveden, Å., Bouchard, C., Carlsson, B., Jacobson, P., Lönroth, H., Maglio, C., Näslund, I., Pirazzi, C., Romeo, S., Sjöholm, K., Sjöström, E., Wedel, H., Svensson, P. A. and Sjöström, L. (2012) 'Bariatric surgery and prevention of type 2 diabetes in Swedish obese subjects'. *The New England Journal of Medicine*, 367: 695–704.

21 Cremieux, P. Y., Buchwald, H., Shikora, S. A., Ghosh, A., Yang, H. E. and Buessing, M. (2008) 'A study on the economic impact of bariatric surgery'. *American Journal of Managed Care*, 14: 589–96.

Chapter Ten: Obesity: The Fears and the Phobias

1 Puhl, R. and Bromwell, K. D. (2001) 'Bias, discrimination and obesity'. *Obesity Research*, 9: 788–805.

2 Latner, J. D. and Stunkard, A. J. (2003) 'Getting worse: the stigmatization of obese children'. *Obesity Research*, 11: 452–6.

3 Fikkan, J. and Rothblum, E. (2005) 'Weight bias in employment', in Brownell, K. D., Puhl, R. M., Schwartz, M. B. and Rudd, L. (eds) *Weight Bias: Nature, Consequence and Remedies*. New York: The Guilford Press: 15–28.

4 Lyons, M. and Ziviani, J. (1995) 'Stereotypes, stigma, and mental illness: learning from fieldwork experiences'. *The American Journal of Occupational Therapy*, 49: 1002–8.

5 Justia US Law (1991) 'Gimello v. Agency Rent-A-Car Systems, Inc.'. Available at: law.justia.com/cases/new-jersey/appellate-division-published/1991/250-n-j-super-338-1.html (Accessed October 2015).

6 Klein, D., Najman, J., Kohrman, A. F. and Munro, C. (1982) 'Patient characteristics that elicit negative responses from family physicians'. *The Journal of Family Practice*, 14: 881–8.

7 Bagley, C. R., Conklin, D. N., Isherwood, R. T., Pechiulis, D. R. and Watson, L. A. (1989) 'Attitudes of nurses toward obesity and obese patients'. *Perceptual and Motor Skills*, 68: 954.

8 Swift, J. A., Hanlon, S., El-Redy, L., Puhl, R. M. and Glazebrook, C. (2013) 'Weight bias among UK trainee dietitians, doctors, nurses and nutritionists'. *Journal of Human Nutrition and Dietetics*, 26: 395–402.

9 Olson, C. L., Schumaker, H. D. and Yawn, B. P. (1994) 'Overweight women delay medical care'. *Archives of Family Medicine*, 3: 888–92.

10 Available at: anred.com.

11 Available at: www.anad.org/get-information/about-eating-disorders/eating-disorders-statistics/

Chapter Eleven: Obesity: Politics, Players and Ploys

1 Haidt, J. (2012) *The Righteous Mind: Why Good People are Divided by Politics and Religion.* London: Penguin.

2 Kahneman, D. (2011) *Thinking Fast and Slow.* London: Penguin Group.

3 Alford, J. R., Funk, C. L. and Hibing, J. R. (2005) 'Are political orientations genetically transmissible'. *American Political Science Review*, 2: 153–67.

4 Pielke, R. A. (2007) *The Honest Broker: Making Sense of Science in Politics.* Cambridge: Cambridge University.

5 Cope, M. B. and Allison, D. B. (2009) 'White hat bias: examples of its presence in obesity research and a call for renewed commitment to faithfulness in research reporting'. *International Journal of Obesity*, 34: 84–8.

6 Cofielda, S. S., Coronab, R. V. and Allison, D. B. (2010) 'Use of causal language in observational studies of obesity and nutrition'. *Obesity Facts*, 3: 353–6.

7 Cope, M. B. and Allison, D. B. (2010) 'White hat bias: examples of its presence in obesity research and a call for renewed commitment to faithfulness in research reporting.' *International Journal of Obesity*, 34 (1): 84–3.

8 Oxman, A. D., Lavis, A. J. N. and Frethem, A. (2007) 'Use of evidence in WHO recommendations'. *Lancet*, 369:1883–9.

9 *Lancet* editorial (2007) 'Science at WHO and UNICEF: the corrosion of trust'. *Lancet*, 370: 1007.

10 Alexander, P. E., Bero, L., Montori, V. M., Brito, J. P., Stoltzfus, R., Djulbegovic, B., Neumann, I., Rave, S. and Guyatt G. (2014) 'World Health Organization recommendations are often strong based on low confidence in effect estimates'. *Journal of Clinical Epidemiology*, 67: 629–34.

11 Alexander, P. E., Brito, J. P., Neumann, I., Gionfriddo, M. R., Bero, L., Djulbegovic, B., Stoltzfus, R., Montori, V. M., Norris, S. L., Schünemann, H. J. and Guyatt, G. H. (2014) 'World Health Organization strong recommendations based on low-quality evidence (study quality) are frequent and often inconsistent with GRADE guidance'. *Journal of Clinical Epidemiology*, 72: 98–106.

12 Kepson, P. (2005) 'Commentary: governance and accountability of NGOs'. *Environmental Science & Policy*, 8: 515–24.

13 PWC (2014) 'The Nature Conservancy: consolidated financial statement'. Available at: nature.org/about-us/our-accountability/annual-report/2014-financial-report-with-report-of-independent-auditors.pdf (Accessed October 2015).

14 BDO (2013) 'World Wildlife Fund, Inc.: financial statements and independent auditor's report'. Available at: assets.worldwildlife.org/financial_reports/23/reports/original/WWF_Non-A133_FS_-_June_03__2014_(S).pdf?1418328169&_ga=1.172723363.1241501934.1443698283 (Accessed October 2015).

15 RSPB (2015) 'Trustees' report and accounts'. Available at: rspb.org.uk/about/run/reportaccounts.aspx (Accessed October 2015).

16 *The Washington Post.* Available at: http://www.washingtonpost.com/wp-dyn/nation/specials/natureconservancy (Accessed October 2015).

17   United States Senate Committee on Finance (2005) 'Grassley statement on committee report on The Nature Conservancy'. Available at:finance.senate.gov/newsroom/chairman/release/?id=d46f51de-oe8b-4d47-b4fa-4f5656codccd (Accesses October 2015).

18   Oxfam 'Behind the Brands'. Available at: behindthebrands.org/en-us/brands (Accessed October 2015).

19   Fooddrink Europe 'Data and trends of the European Food and Drink Industry 2013–2014'. Available at: fooddrinkeurope.eu/uploads/publications_documents/Data_Trends_of_the_European_Food_and_Drink_Industry_2013-20141.pdf (Accessed October 2015).

Chapter Twelve: Weight Management: The Personal Perspective

1   Tsuneo Nishiaw, T., Akaoka, L., Nishida, Y., Kawaguchi, Y., Hayashi, E. and Takashi Yoshimura, T. (1976) 'Some factors related to obesity in the Japanese sumo wrestler'. *American Journal of Clinical Nutrition*, 29: 1167–74.

2   Simmons, A. M. (1998) 'Where fat is a mark of beauty'. *Los Angeles Times*. Available at: anthroprof.org/documents/Docs102/102articles/fat26.pdf (Accessed October 2015).

3   'Actors who have gained or lost weight for film roles, in pictures'. *The Daily Telegraph*. Available at: telegraph.co.uk/culture/culturepicturegalleries/10238141/Actors-who-have-gained-or-lost-weight-for-film-roles.html?frame=3074658 (Accessed October 2015).

4   Henry, C. (2005) 'Basal metabolic rate studies in humans: measurement and development of new equations'. *Public Health Nutrition*, 8: 1,133–52.

5   Council of Scientific Affairs of the American Medical Association (1988) 'Treatment of obesity in adults'. *JAMA*, 260: 2547–1551.

6   Foxcroft, L. (2011) *Calories and Corsets: A History of Dieting over 2,000 Years*. London: Profile Books.

7   Sacks, F. M., Bray, G. A., Carey, V. J., Smith, S. R., Anton, S. D., McManus, K., Champagne, C. M., Bishop, L. M., Laranjo, N., Meryl, S. L. et al. (2009) 'Comparison of weight-loss diets with different compositions of fat, protein, and carbohydrates'. *The New England Medical Journal*, 360: 859–73.

8   Johnston, B. C., Kanters, S., Bandayrel, K., Wu, P., Naji, F., Siemieniuk, R. A., Ball, G. D., Busse, J. W., Thorlund, K., Guyatt, G. et al. (2014) 'Comparison of weight loss among named diet programs in overweight and obese adults: a meta-analysis'. *JAMA*, 312: 923–33.

9   European Food Safety Authority (2010) 'Scientific opinion on the substantiation of health claims related to conjugated linoleic acid (CLA) isomers and contribution to the maintenance or achievement of a normal body weight (ID 686, 726, 1516, 1518, 2892, 3165), increase in lean body mass (ID 498, 731), increase in insulin sensitivity (ID 1517), protection of DNA, proteins and lipids from oxidative damage (ID 564, 1937), and contribution to immune defences by stimulation of production of protective antibodies in response to vaccination (ID 687, 1519) pursuant to Article 13(1) of Regulation (EC) No 1924/2006'. *EFSA Journal*, 8 (10): 1794.

10   Wansink, B. (2010) *Mindless Eating: Why We Eat More than We Think*. London: Hay House.

11   Rolls, B. (2012) *The Ultimate Volumetrics Diet*. New York: Harper Collins.

12 Rolls, B. J., Bell, E. A. and Thorwart, M. L. (1999) 'Water incorporated into a food but not served with a food decreases energy intake in lean women'. *American Journal of Clinical Nutrition*, 4: 448–55.

13 Leahy, K. E., Birch, L. L. and Rolls, B. J. (2008) 'Reducing the energy density of multiple meals decreases the energy intake of preschool-age children'. *American Journal of Clinical Nutrition*, 6: 1459–68.

14 Ledikwe, J. H., Rolls, B. J., Smiciklas-Wright, H., Mitchell, D. C., Ard, J. D., Champagne, C., Karanja, N., Lin, P. H., Stevens, V. J. and Appel, L. J. (2007) 'Reductions in dietary energy density are associated with weight loss in overweight and obese participants in the PREMIER trial'. *American Journal of Clinical Nutrition*, 85: 1212–21.

15 Hill, J. O., Peters, J. C. and Jortberg, J. (2004) *The Step Diet*. New York: Workman Publishing.

Chapter Thirteen: Weight Management: The National Perspective

1 Eskes, T. K. (2000) 'From anemia to spina bifida – the story of folic acid. A tribute to Professor Richard Smithells'. *European Journal of Obstetrics, Gynecology, and Reproductive Biology*, 90: 119–23.

2 Kahneman, D. (2011) *Thinking Fast and Slow*. London: Penguin Group.

3 Nuffield Council on Bioethics (2007) *Public Health: Ethical Issues*. Cambridge: Nuffield Council on Bioethics. Available at: nuffieldbioethics.org/wp-content/uploads/2014/07/Public-health-ethical-issues.pdf (Accessed October 2015).

4 Nielson (2015) 'We are what we eat: healthy eating trends around the world'. Available at: nielsen.com/content/dam/nielsenglobal/eu/nielseninsights/pdfs/Nielsen%20Global%20Health%20and%20Wellness%20Report%20-%20January%202015.pdf (Accessed October 2015).

5 Centers for Disease Control and Prevention (2014) 'Perception of weight status in US children and adolescents aged 8–15 years, 2005–2012'. Available at: cdc.gov/nchs/data/databriefs/db158.htm (Accessed October 2015).

6 http://www.mckinsey.com/industries/healthcare-systems-and-services/our-insights/how-the-world-could-better-fight-obesity (Accessed October 2015).

7 Mattes, R. (2014) 'Energy intake and obesity: ingestive frequency outweighs portion size'. *Physiology & Behavior*, 134: 110–18.

8 Walters, J. (2015) 'Burger King eliminates soft drinks from children's meal menus'. *The Guardian*. Available at:theguardian.com/society/2015/mar/10/burger-king-soft-drinks-childrens-menu (Accessed October 2015).

9 Hanks, A. S., Just, D. R. and Wansink, B. (2014) 'Chocolate milk consequences: a pilot study evaluating the consequences of banning chocolate milk in school cafeterias'. *PLOS One*, 9 (4): e91022.

10 Dwyer, J. T., Michell, P., Cosentino, C., Webber, L., Seed, J. M., Hoelscher, D., Snyder, M. P., Stevens, M. and Nader, P. (2003) 'Fat-sugar see-saw in school lunches: impact of a low fat intervention'. *Journal of Adolescent Health*, 32 (6): 428–35.

11 Irish Universities Nutrition Alliance (2011) 'National Adult Nutrition Survey'. Available at: iuna.net/?p=106 (Accessed October 2015).

12 Briggs, A. D. M., Mytton, O. T., Madden, D., O'Shea, D., Rayner, M. and Scarborough, P. (2015) 'The potential impact on obesity of a 10% tax on sugar-sweetened beverages in Ireland, an effect assessment modeling study'. *BMC Public Health*, 13: 860–9.

13 Madden, D. (2015) 'The poverty effects of a "fat-tax" in Ireland'. *Health Economics*, 24: 104–21.

14 FBI report (2015) 'Ring leaders plead guilty in $20 Million WIC and food stamp fraud conspiracy'. Available at: fbi.gov/atlanta/press-releases/2015/ring-leaders-plead-guilty-in-20-million-wic-and-food-stamp-fraud-conspiracy (Accessed October 2015).

Chapter Fourteen: The Way Forward

1 Foresight (2010) *Tackling Obesities: Future Choices – Project Report*. London: Government Office of Science.

2 Swinburn, B., Kraak, V., Rutter, H., Vandevijvere, S., Lobstein, T., Sacks, G., Gomes, F., Marsh, T. and Magnusson, R. (2015) 'Strengthening of accountability systems to create healthy food environments and reduce global obesity. *Lancet*, 385: 2534–45.

3 Lobstein, T. and Davies, S. (2009) 'Defining and labelling "healthy" and "unhealthy" food'. *Public Health Nutrition*, 12: 331–40.

4 Sinclair, S. E., Cooper, M. and Mansfield, E. D. (2014) 'The influence of menu labeling on calories selected or consumed: a systematic review and meta-analysis'. *Journal of the Academy of Nutrition and Dietetics*, 114: 1375–88.

5 Hollands, G. J., Shemilt, I., Marteau, T. M., Jebb, S. A., Lewis, H. B., Wei, Y., Higgins, J. P. T. and Ogilvie, D. (2015) 'Portion, package or tableware size for changing selection and consumption of food, alcohol and tobacco'. *Cochrane Database of Systematic Reviews*, 9: CD011045. DOI: 10.1002/14651858.CD011045.pub2.

6 Gornall, J. (2015) 'Sugar: spinning a web of influence'. *BMJ*, 350: h231. doi: 10.1136/bmj.h231.

7 Heude, B., Kattaneh, A., Rakotovao, R., Bresson, J. L., Boys, J. M., Ducimetière, P. and Charles, M. A. (2005) 'Anthropometric relationships between parents and children throughout childhood: the Fleurbaix-Laventie Ville Santé Study'. *International Journal of Obesity*, 29: 1222–9.

8 EPODE (Ensemble Prévenons l'Obesité Des Enfants – Together Let's prevent childhood obesity). http://epode-international-network.com/

Index

Topic: Interpersonal Skills   **Subtopic:** Empathy

Notes to Parents and Teachers:

As a child becomes more familiar reading books, it is important for them to rely on and use reading strategies more independently to help figure out words they do not know.

REMEMBER: PRAISE IS A GREAT MOTIVATOR!

Here are some praise points for beginning readers:

• I saw you get your mouth ready to say the first letter of that word.
• I like the way you used the picture to help you figure out that word.
• I noticed that you saw some sight words you knew how to read!

Book Ends for the Reader!

Here are some reminders before reading the text:

• Point to each word you read to make it match what you say.

• Use the picture for help.

• Look at and say the first letter sound of the word.

• Look for sight words that you know how to read in the story.

• Think about the story to see what word might make sense.

Words to Know Before You Read

beach

build

favorite

merman

noises

quiet

turtle

water

How to Be
Friends with This Merman

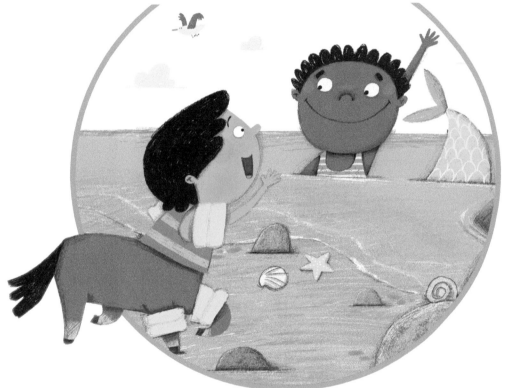

By Erin Savory
Illustrated by Ana Zurita

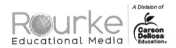
Rourke
Educational Media

A Division of
Carson Dellosa
Education.

I met Milo at the beach.

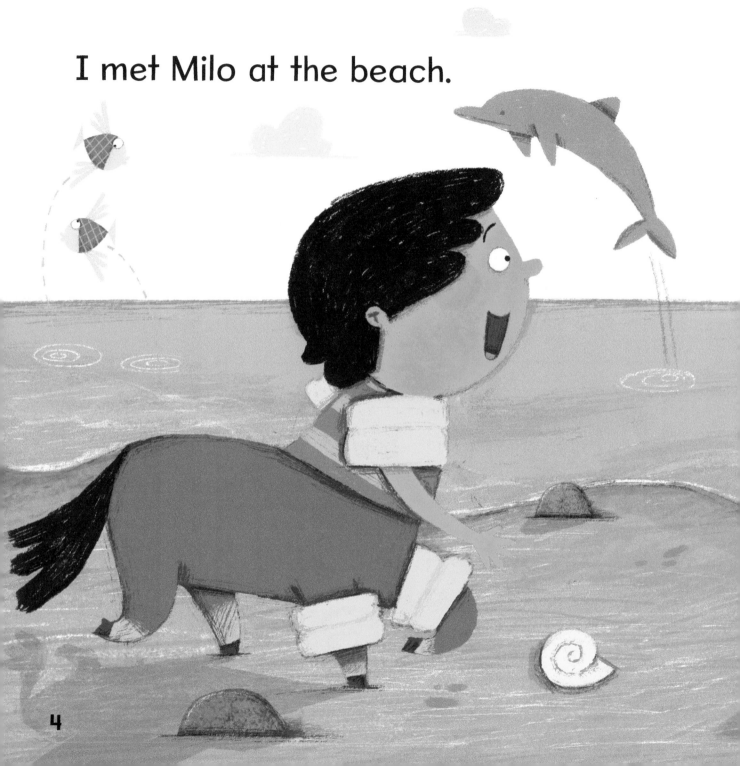

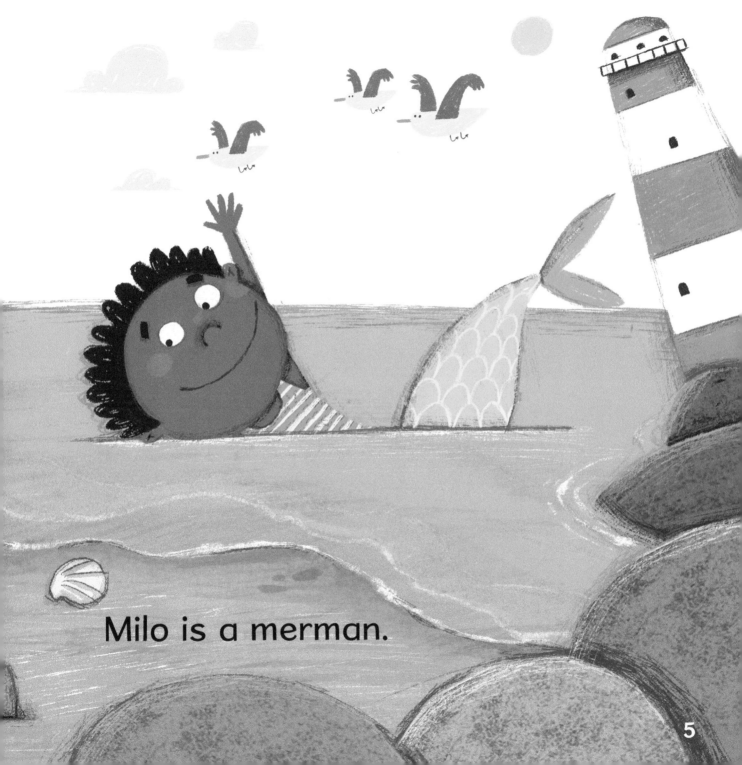

Milo is a merman.

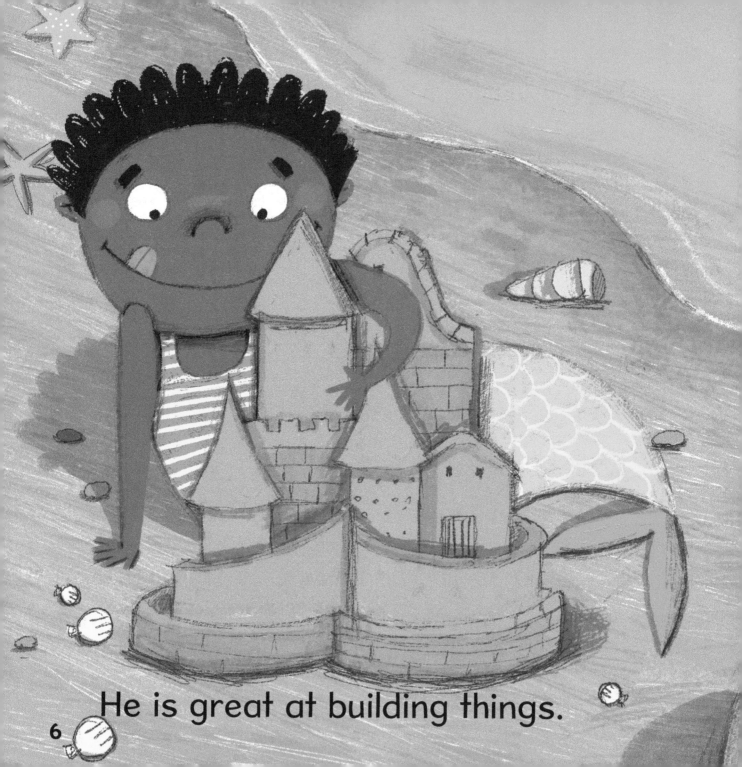

He is great at building things.

6

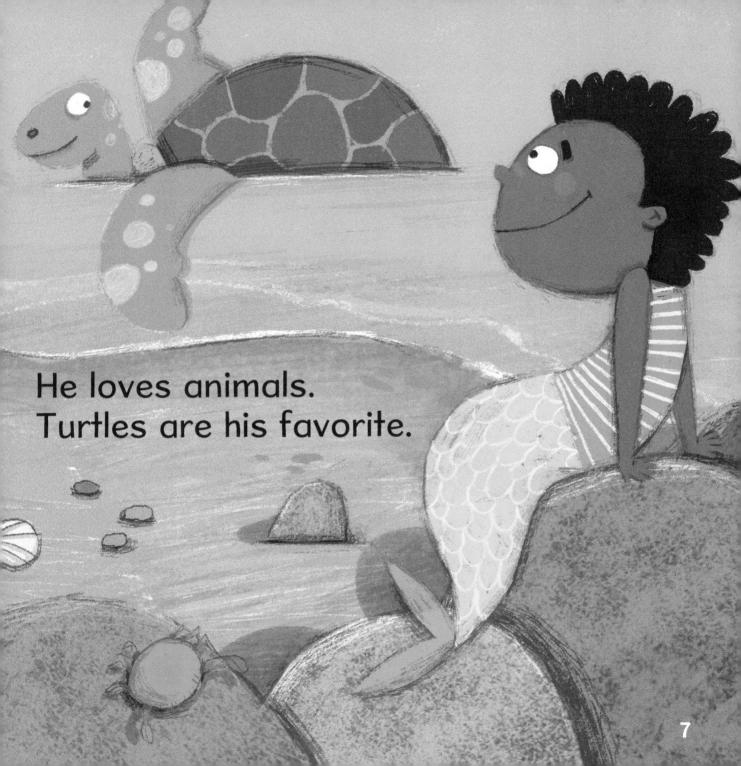

He loves animals.
Turtles are his favorite.

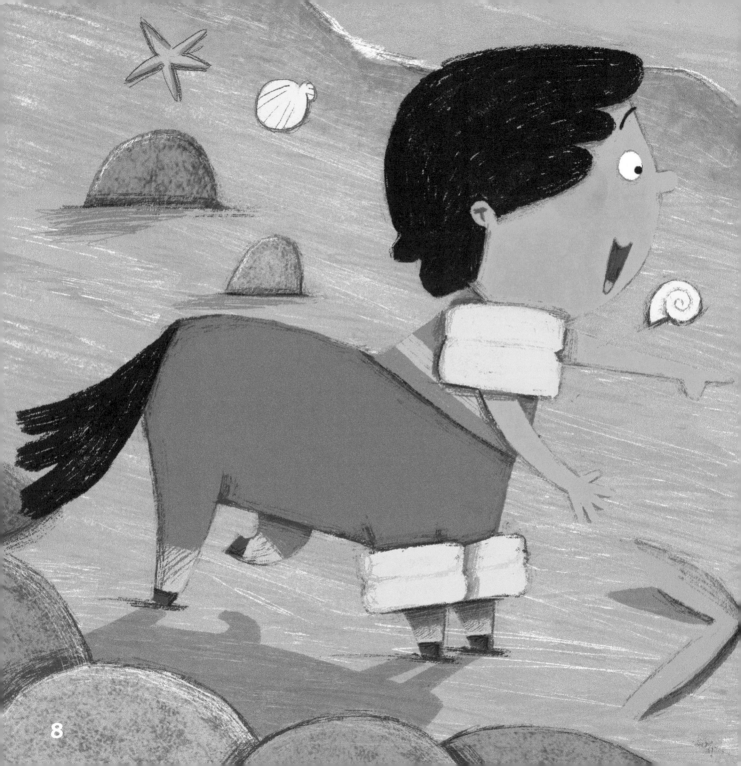

8

How can I be friends
with this merman?

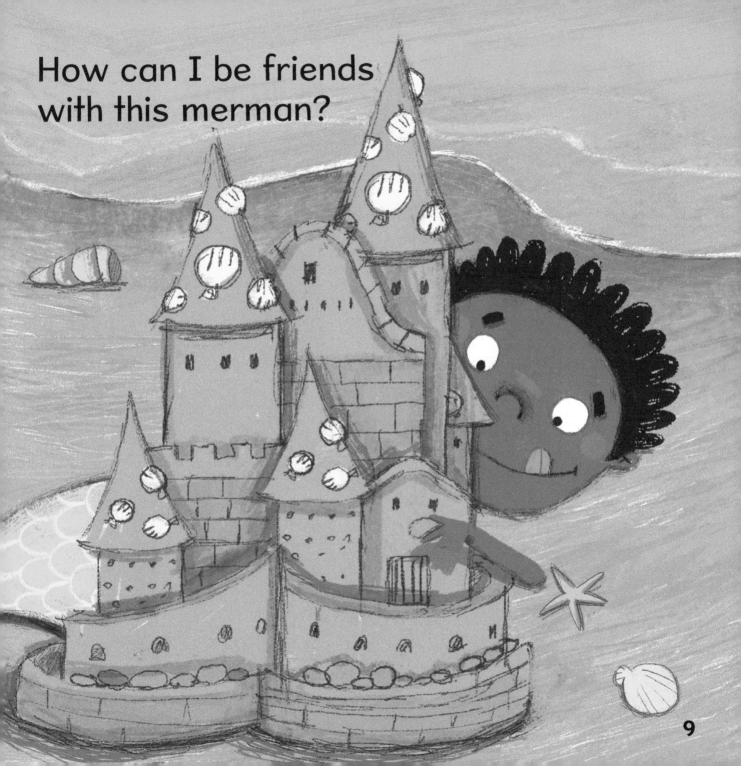

I build with him.

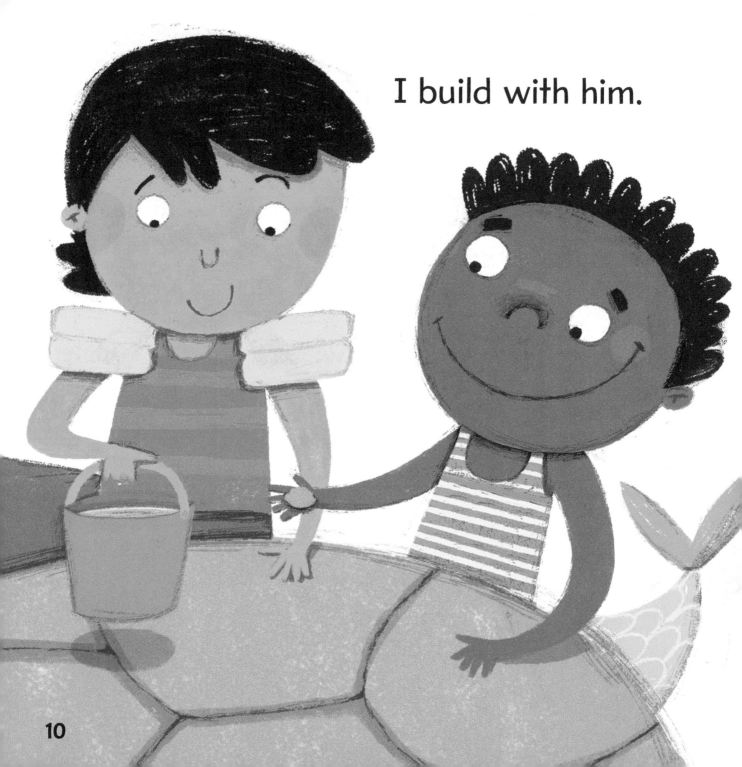

He teaches me new things.

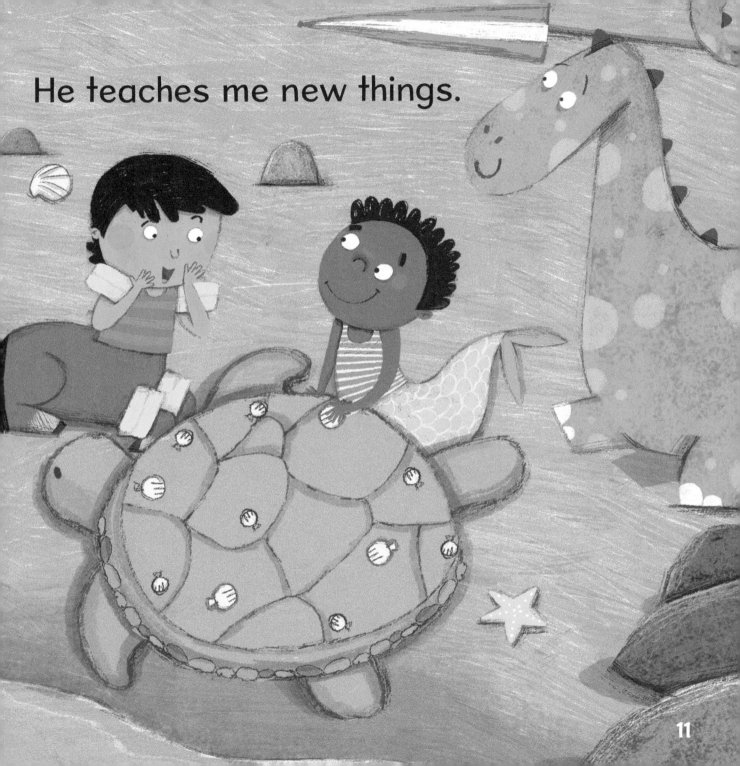

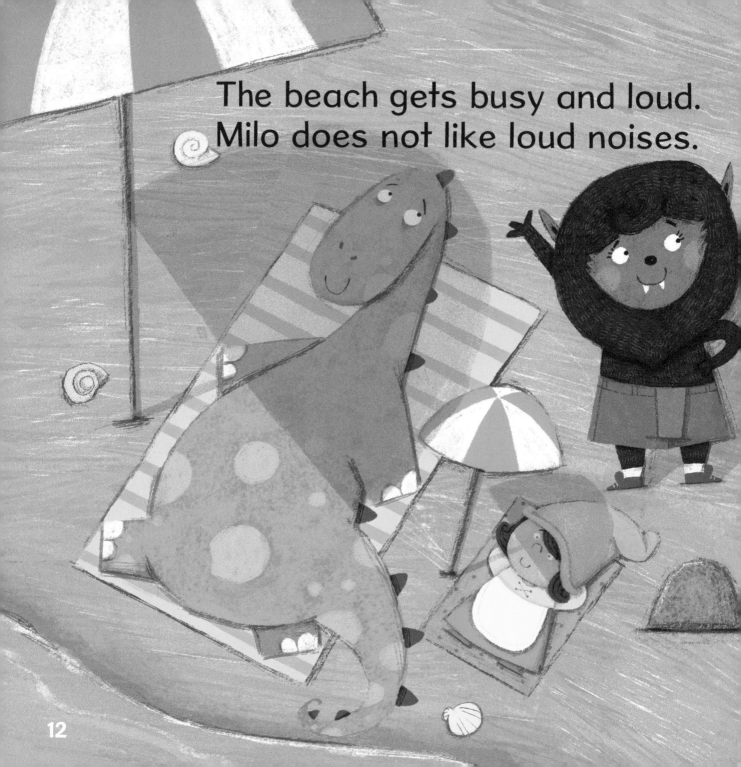

The beach gets busy and loud.
Milo does not like loud noises.

12

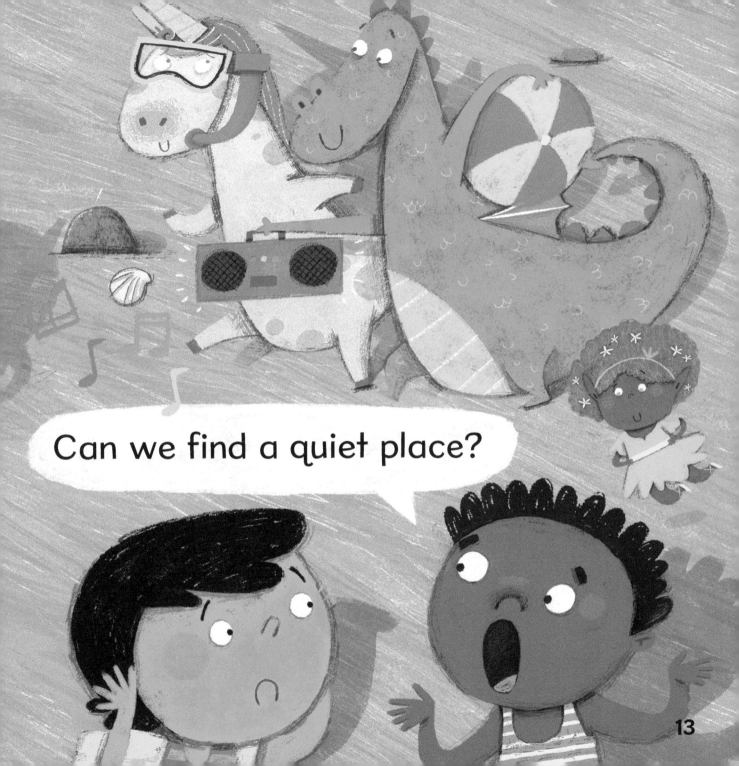

13

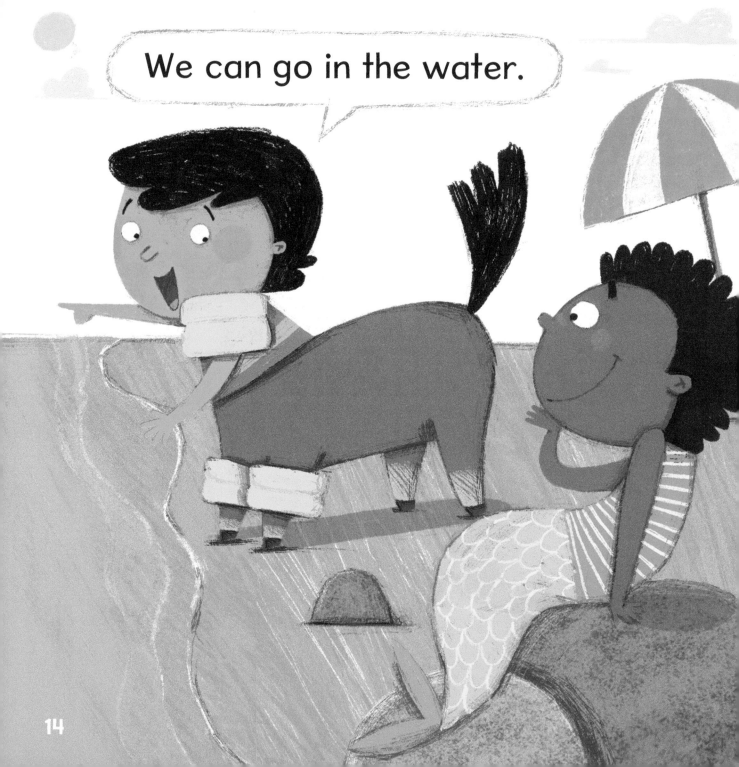

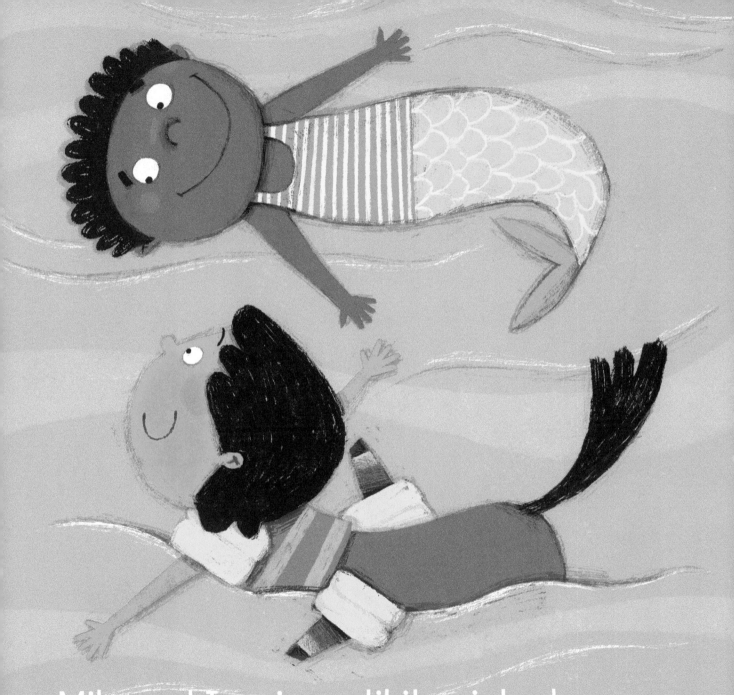

Milo and I swim until it quiets down.

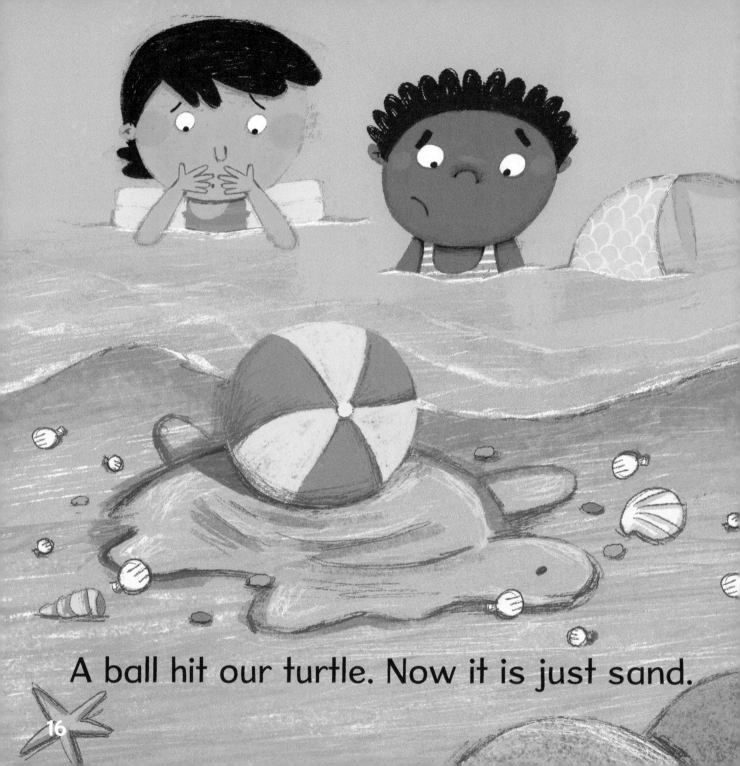

A ball hit our turtle. Now it is just sand.

16

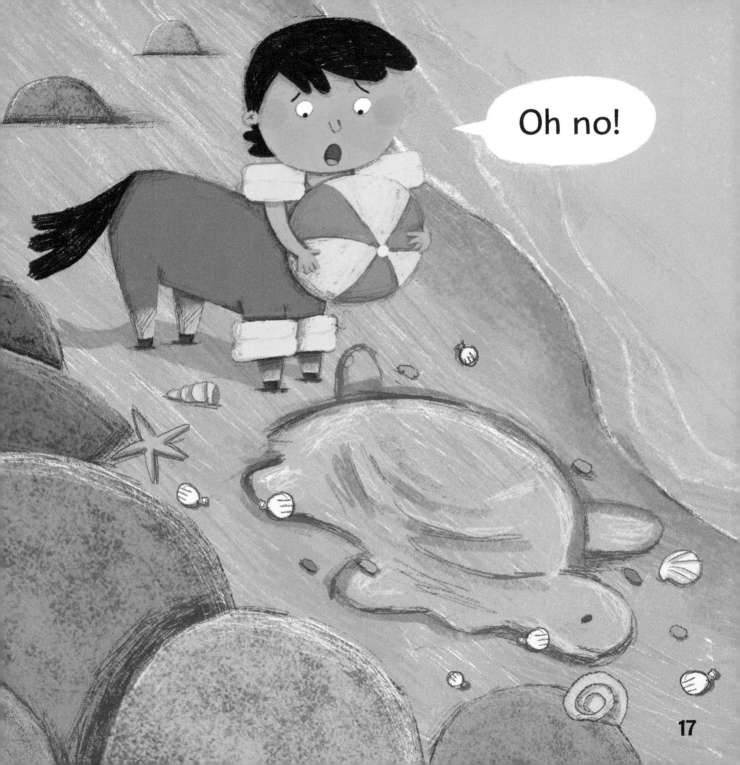

17

Milo cheers me up.

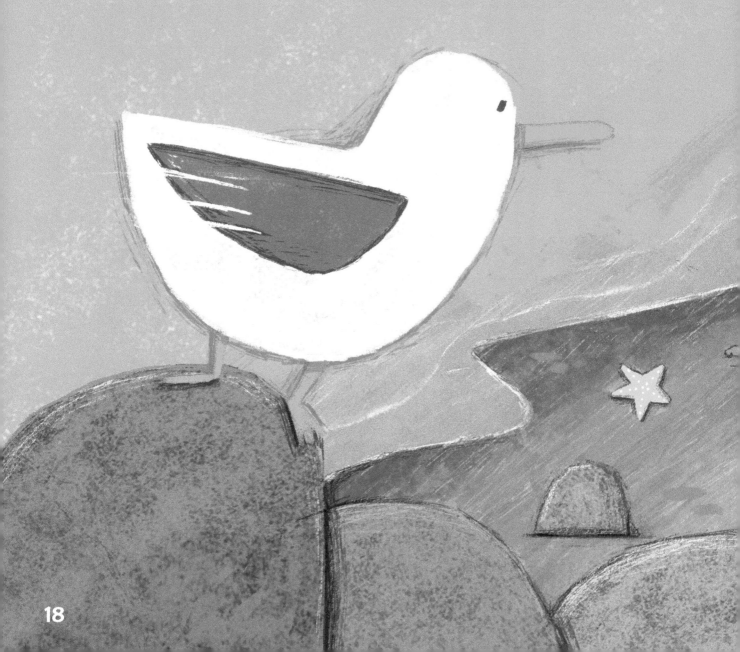

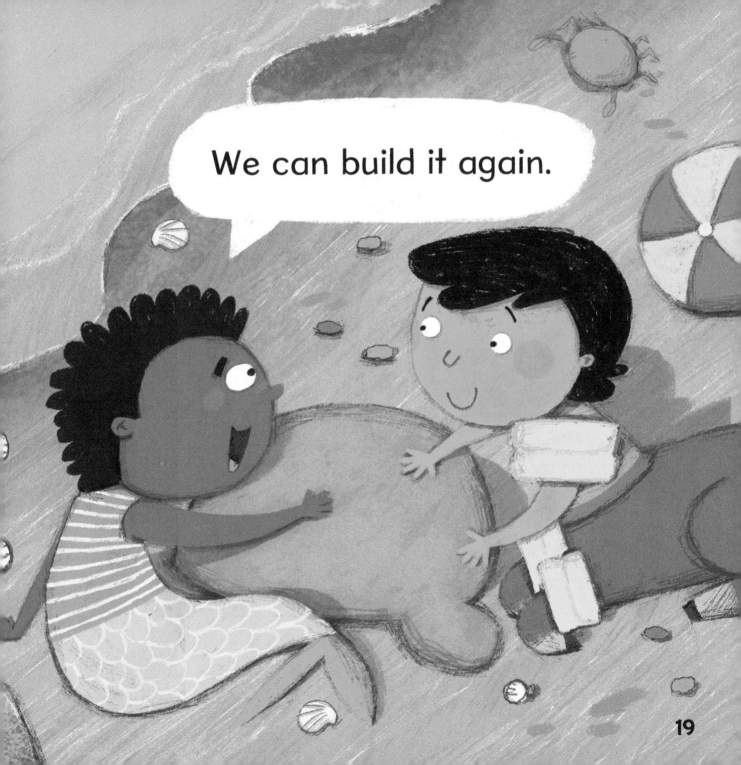

19

How can you be friends with
this merman?

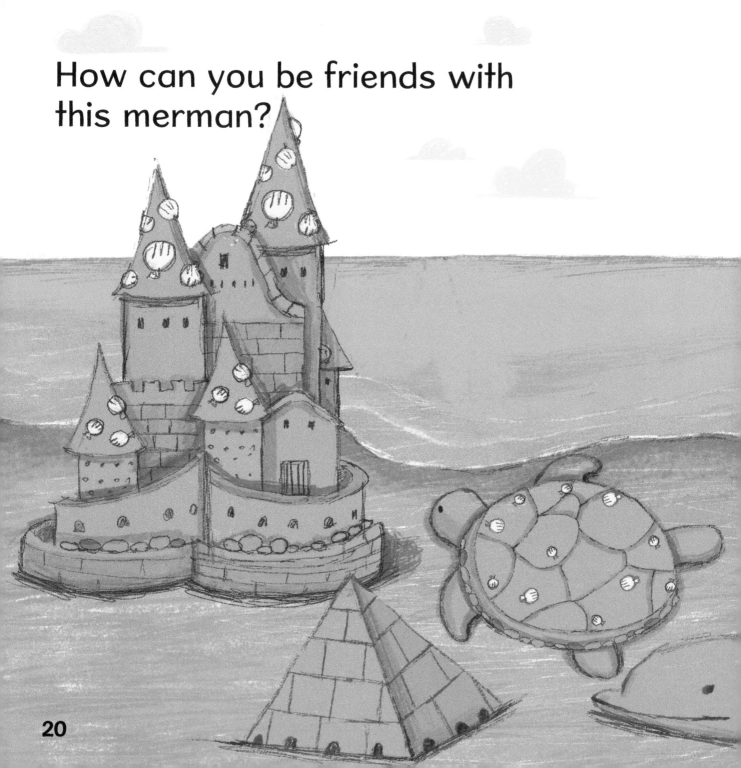

20

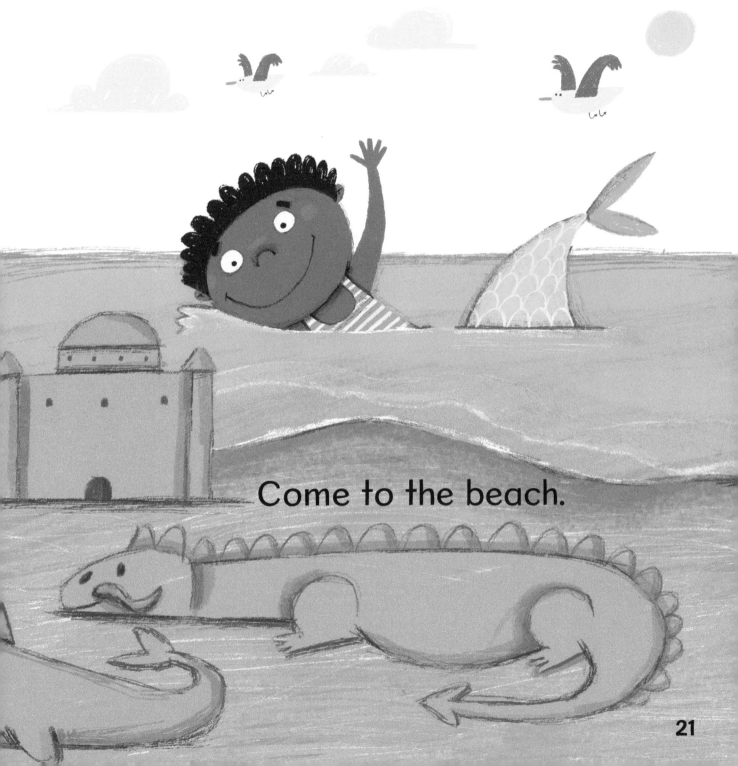

Come to the beach.

21

Milo will be happy to meet you!

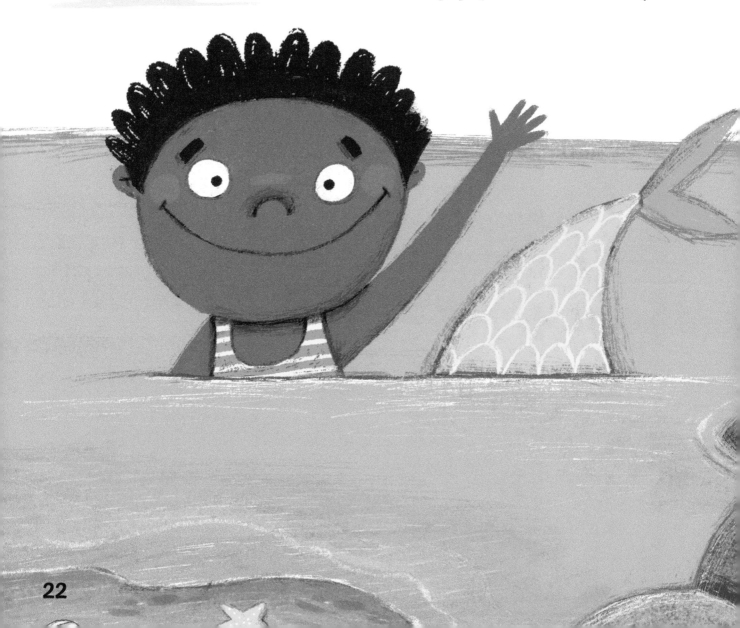

Book Ends for the Reader

"I know..."
What does Milo like to do?

"I think..."
How do you feel when you hear loud noises?

What happened in this book?
Look at each picture and talk about what happened in the story.

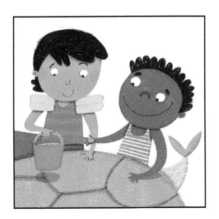
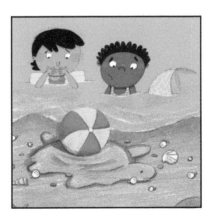

About the Author

Erin Savory is a writer who lives in Florida. She loves to paint with her two-year-old son. She loves spending time in nature. Reading is her favorite activity.

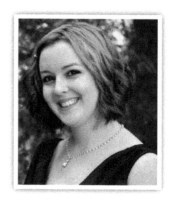

About the Illustrator

Ana Zurita was born by the sea in Valencia, Spain, where she completed her studies in Fine Arts and currently lives with her wonderful family. She is a big fan of the beach in winter, the color yellow, the smell of old books, and heavy blankets. But what has made her the happiest from a very early age is drawing. That's why her greatest dream is to make others happy with her illustrations.

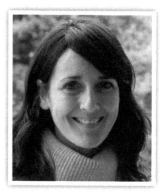

Library of Congress PCN Data

How to Be Friends with This Merman / Erin Savory
(How to Be Friends)
 ISBN 978-1-73164-346-9 (hard cover)(alk. paper)
 ISBN 978-1-73164-310-0 (soft cover)
 ISBN 978-1-73164-378-0 (e-Book)
 ISBN 978-1-73164-410-7 (ePub)
Library of Congress Control Number: 2020945145

Rourke Educational Media

01-3502011937

www.rourkeeducationalmedia.com

Edited by: Tracie Santos
Layout by: Morgan Burnside
Cover and interior illustrations by: Ana Zurita

CPSIA information can be obtained
at www.ICGtesting.com
Printed in the USA
BVHW060718210522
637336BV00001B/10

9 781731 643100